100 Questions & Answers
About Sleep and
Sleep Disorders

Second Edition

Edison, NJ

World Headquarters

Jones and Bartlett Publishers	Jones and Bartlett Publishers	Jones and Bartlett Publishers
40 Tall Pine Drive	Canada	International
Sudbury, MA 01776	6339 Ormindale Way	Barb House, Barb Mews
978-443-5000	Mississauga, Ontario L5V 1J2	London W6 7PA
info@jbpub.com	Canada	United Kingdom
www.jbpub.com		

Jones and Bartlett's books and products are available through most bookstores and online book-sellers. To contact Jones and Bartlett Publishers directly, call 800-832-0034, fax 978-443-8000, or visit our website, www.jbpub.com.

Substantial discounts on bulk quantities of Jones and Bartlett's publications are available to corporations, professional associations, and other qualified organizations. For details and specific discount information, contact the special sales department at Jones and Bartlett via the above contact information or send an email to specialsales@jbpub.com.

Production Credits

Executive Publisher: Christopher Davis
Associate Editor: Kathy Richardson
Production Director: Amy Rose
Production Editor: Daniel Stone
Associate Marketing Manger: Rebecca Wasley
V.P. of Manufacturing and
   Inventory Control: Therese Connell
Composition: Auburn Associates, Inc.
Cover Design: Jonathan Ayotte
Printing and Binding: Malloy, Inc.
Cover Printing: Malloy, Inc.

Photo Credits

Top Left: © Victoria Alexandrova/Shutterstock, Inc.
Bottom Left: © JDP Productions/Shutterstock, Inc.
Top Right: © Thierry Maffeis/Shutterstock, Inc.
Bottom Right: © Karen Winton/Shutterstock, Inc.

Library of Congress Cataloging-in-Publication Data
Chokroverty, Sudhansu.
   100 questions & answers about sleep and sleep disorders / Sudhansu Chokroverty.
     p. cm.
   Rev. ed. of: 100 questions about sleep and sleep disorders. 2001.
   Includes index.
   ISBN-13: 978-0-7637-4120-4
   ISBN-10: 0-7637-4120-5
   1. Sleep disorders—Miscellanea. 2. Sleep—Miscellanea. I. 100 questions about sleep and sleep disorders. II. Title. III. Title: One hundred questions and answers about sleep and sleep disorders.
   RC547.C483 2008
   616.8'498—dc22

2007030439

6048

Printed in the United States of America
11 10 09 08 07   10 9 8 7 6 5 4 3 2 1

Contents

Part 2: Risk/Prevention/Epidemiology 27

Part 3: Diagnosis 47

Part 4: Treatment — 85

Part 5: Living with a Sleep Disorder   109

Contents

vii

Acknowledgments

It is my great pleasure to express my gratitude and appreciation to my wife, Manisha Chokroverty, MD, for her forbearance and unfailing support during the preparation of this book, including this revision, and for suggesting some of the questions in this monograph.

I would like to thank Mark Mahowald, MD, for reviewing the first edition of this book and for providing thoughtful and insightful comments.

I would like to thank Betty Coram for typing and Sara Sowers for editing and making corrections. I must thank Christopher Davis, Executive Publisher, Medicine at Jones and Bartlett Publishers for his thoughtfulness and professionalism. I would also like to thank Kathy Richardson, Associate Editor at Jones and Bartlett Publishers, for her help in publishing the book. Finally, I must thank my numerous patients who, over the years, have taught me the value of listening to them in order to learn real sleep medicine, which cannot be mastered by only reading books.

Sleep has fascinated mankind since time immemorial. This interest has been reflected in the writings of poets, philosophers, and scientists alike. In the second half of the last century, significant developments took place in our understanding of sleep. Public awareness about the importance of a good night's sleep is now increasing, thanks to the efforts of the American Academy of Sleep Medicine, other scientific organizations (such as the Sleep Section of the American Academy of Neurology and the American Thoracic Society), National Sleep Foundation, and print and broadcast media.

Why should we be interested in knowing about sleep? Some fundamental facts about the magnitude of the problem go a long way toward answering this question. According to a National Commission for Sleep Disorders Research (NCSDR) report published in 1993, approximately 40 million Americans suffer from chronic disorders of sleep and wakefulness. The vast majority of these individuals remain undiagnosed and untreated by the medical community, contributing to expenses that are measured in terms of billions of dollars. An additional 20 to 30 million people experience intermittent sleep problems. Several recent surveys have revealed that one-third of Americans suffer from sleeplessness; in 10 percent of these individuals, the problem is a persistent one. The Department of Transportation estimates that 200,000 automobile accidents each year may be sleep-related. In a 1995 Gallup survey, one-third of adults admitted to having dozed off while driving a car.

Other startling statistics have been gathered about sleep disorders. For example, an estimated 25 to 30 million Americans suffer from chronic insomnia, and 15 to 20 million suffer from sleep apnea. In an important study from Wisconsin, 4 percent of men and 2 percent of women between 30 and 60 years of age were found to have sleep apnea. Five million Americans suffer from sleep disorders due to shift work. More than 250,000 Americans have narcolepsy, a disorder of excessive sleepiness.

Several national and international disasters can also be cited to illustrate the magnitude of sleep-related problems. A number of catastrophes are thought to be related to fatigue and sleepiness, including the *Exxon Valdes* oil spill in Alaska; the nuclear-near disaster at Three Mile Island, Pennsylvania; the nuclear accident at Chernobyl in the former Soviet Union; the Bhopal (India) gas leak disaster, which killed nearly 20,000 people; and the *Challenger* space shuttle disaster.

It is, therefore, imperative for both the public and members of the healthcare profession to be aware of the importance of a good night's sleep and sleep problems. This book of 100 questions will cover various aspects of normal and abnormal sleep that are of practical relevance.

PART ONE

The Basics

1. What is sleep?

Since the dawn of civilization, all the movers, shakers and thinkers of the world, the philosophers, religious scholars, scientists and poets have been asking this question without any satisfactory answer. More realistically and correctly this question should be asked when one is trying to get to sleep. But then it is difficult to ask this question when we lie down, close our eyes and try to forget about the world of wakefulness. Slowly, we begin drifting into a state beyond wakefulness when we do not see, hear or perceive things in a rational or logical manner. We are in another world where we have no control, our brain cannot respond logically and adequately and our body is relatively immobile. We are now entering what is termed "**predormitum**". Soon, we are drifting from lighter to deeper stages of sleep. We are now unconscious. Fortunately, this state is reversible—a characteristic that differentiates sleep from irreversible coma (complete unconsciousness as a result of a disease) and death. We will wake up to see the world of wakefulness after seven to eight hours of sleep. Most of us today go to sleep at night (unless you are working a night shift). We finish our day's activities and after relaxing in the evening, we prepare to go to sleep. It is interesting to note as Roger Ekirch wrote in his fascinating book called *At Day's Close* that centuries before the discovery of light and electricity nocturnal sleep habits of humankind were different from the consolidated sleep we seek nowadays. In the days past, there were 2 periods of sleep at night consisting of 4 hours at a stretch with a break of 2 to 3 hours in between. This interval period was occupied by mankind for future planning, dreaming, meditating and visiting.

Predormitum

A state of diminished perception and control through which a person passes in progressing from wakefulness into the sleep state.

Centuries before the discovery of light and electricity nocturnal sleep habits of humankind were different from the consolidated sleep we seek nowadays.

Sleep is not simply an absence of wakefulness and perception—it is not just a passive phenomenon resulting from withdrawal of all sensory stimuli. Many areas of the brain remain active during sleep. Both passive mechanisms (for example, withdrawal of all external and internal stimulation) and active mechanisms contribute to sleep. All of the mechanisms responsible for generating sleep are located within the brain. Indeed, this function of the brain contributes to the individual's overall health, affecting not only the brain but also the entire body as evidenced by the many diseases resulting from too much sleep, too little sleep, inappropriate timing of sleep, or abnormal movements and behavior intruding into sleep.

Modern sleep scientists define sleep based on the behavior of the person while asleep and the physiological changes that occur in the waking brain as one is drifting into sleep. The behavioral criteria include a characteristic posture, relative immobility, impaired response to external stimulation, and closed eyes. The physiologic criteria define the various sleep stages and are based on recordings of electrical activities of the brain (**electroencephalogram, or EEG**), the muscles (**electromyogram, or EMG**), and eye movement (**electrooculogram, or EOG**).

We divide sleep broadly into two states: **non-rapid eye movement (NREM) sleep** and **rapid eye movement (REM) sleep**. Thus we exist in three states—wakefulness, NREM, and REM sleep with different controls and functions.

NREM sleep is traditionaly further divided into four stages which have been slightly modified in a recent revision combining traditional stages 3 and 4 into stage N3

Many areas of the brain remain active during sleep.

The Basics

Electroencephalogram (EEG)

Recording of the electrical activities of the brain.

Electromyogram (EMG)

Recording of the electrical activities of the muscles.

Electro-oculogram (EOG)

Recording of the movements of the eye.

We exist in three states—wakefulness, NREM, and REM sleep with different controls and functions.

NREM

Non-rapid eye movement sleep. Multistage phase of the progression from wakefulness into deep sleep.

REM

Rapid eye movement sleep. The stage of sleep during which dreaming occurs.

only. In stage 1, the predominant wakeful brain rhythms of an adult decrease to less than half of those seen in the wakeful state, the muscle tone decreases a little, and some rolling, slow eye movements take place. In stage 2 NREM sleep, brain electrical activities show a characteristic pattern, called **sleep spindles** (brain rhythms of 14 to 16 cycles per second that are seen in surface recordings taken from the front and center of the head); the sleep spindles are accompanied by slower waves (less than 4 cycles per second) during less than 20 percent of the time. The slow-wave or deep sleep, which is a combination of traditional stages 3 and 4 or the recent revision called stage N3, is dominated by brain waves slower than 4 cycles per second. Most of our time during sleep is spent in stage 2 NREM sleep.

Sleep spindles

Brain rhythms of 14 to 16 cycles per second thast are seen in surface recordings taken from the front and center of the head during NREM sleep.

There is an orderly pro-gression of sleep pattern in a normal adult human being.

There is an orderly progression of sleep pattern in a normal adult human being. Approximately 5 to 10 minutes after sleep onset, we drift from stage 1 to stage 2 and then in about 1 hour, we go into slow-wave sleep. Roughly 60 to 90 minutes after sleep onset, we enter into the world of dream sleep—that is, REM sleep, the stage in which most dreams occur. Eyeballs move rapidly under the closed eyelids (hence the name "rapid eye movement sleep"). Muscle tone in the EMG recording decreases markedly or is absent and the brain waves (EEG) resemble those noted during wakefulness. NREM and REM sleep alternate in a cyclical manner (about 4 to 6 cycles) interspersed with brief periods of wakefulness throughout the night. During the first third of the night, slow-wave sleep dominates; conversely, during the last third of the night, REM sleep dominates. REM sleep accounts for 20 to 25% of the sleep period.

REM sleep accounts for 20 to 25% of the sleep period.

Different sleep patterns, including the time occupied by different stages of sleep, are observed in newborns, children and the elderly (see Question 12).

2. Why do we sleep?

The proper question is "do we need sleep and can we get by without sleep?" The answer is definitely in the negative because if we do not have adequate sleep at night, we feel sleepy, irritable and awful throughout the day. Again, this question of the function of sleep has been debated throughout the centuries without an adequate answer. According to some recent evidence, both the brain and the rest of the body need an optimal amount of sleep. Although the exact function of sleep is not known, several theories have been proposed based on the results of animal and human sleep deprivation experiments. For example, we may require sleep for energy conservation and for restoration of the body and brain that allows them to function adequately during the wakeful period. It has been suggested that sleep is needed for both consolidation and reconsolidation of memory (restoration of lost memory after the period of sleep) and for adequate stimulation of various nerve circuits within the brain that ensure its proper functioning. Recent evidence also suggests that different genes (expression of proteins) are transcripted in the brain during sleep and wakefulness indicating different functions of the brain during these two states. In addition, sleep may provide for regulation of body temperature. Although we do not know its exact functions, sleep is critical for our survival and for maintaining good physical and mental health.

3. What is my sleep requirement?

The average requirement for a normal adult man or woman is approximately 7½ to 8 hours.

Human sleep requirements vary depending on a person's age. The average requirement for a normal adult man or woman is approximately 7½ to 8 hours. Sleep requirements, just like many behavioral functions and requirements, assume a bell-shaped curve, however. Thus some people require less than the average amount of sleep and some require more sleep to function adequately during waking hours. Some individuals can get by with 6 to 7 hours of sleep (or less); others require 9 to 10 hours of sleep each night. It is important to emphasize the misperception that many people may have, especially those who suffer from insomnia, that everyone must have 7½ to 8 hours of sleep or he/she will not be able to function during the daytime. Your sleep requirement is the amount of sleep you need to feel rested, refreshed and energetic on awakening in the morning and, therefore, ready to function adequately. The basic sleep requirement is defined by heredity rather than by any environmental influence.

The basic sleep requirement is defined by heredity rather than by any environmental influence.

4. How does sunrise or sunset control when we sleep and wake up?

Our sleep-wake habits are controlled not only by external light and darkness as determined by sunrise and sunset, but also by our internal body clock. This question was first raised more than two and a half centuries ago by a French astronomer named de Mairin. He noticed that the leaves of a heliotrope plant would open at sunrise and close at sunset, even when the plant was kept inside away from sunlight. This observation led de Mairin to conclude that an internal clock in the plant must control the opening and closing of the leaves. Only in 1980 did scientists discover the existence of an internal clock in rats. Shortly thereafter, researchers confirmed that such a clock operates in humans as well.

The human internal clock is thought to reside within a cluster of nerve cells (called **suprachiasmatic nuclei**) located deep in the center of the brain above the **pituitary gland**, the organ that is responsible for secretion of several important hormones. The paired suprachiasmatic nuclei are part of the **hypothalamus**, which controls the secretion of the hormones, food and water intake, body temperature, emotion, and sleep-wake regulation. These nerve cells are located above the crossing pathways that transmit signals from **retina** (the layer of nerve cells in the back of the eye responsible for transmitting visual images) to the back of the brain. This internal clock has widespread connections— not only with the retina for receiving light from the outside world, but also with other parts of the nervous system. As a result, it controls the body's sleep-wake cycle, secretion of hormones, and the body's temperature rhythms.

Every living cell has a rhythm. For example, our sleep-wake habit follows a **circadian** (from the Latin *circa*, meaning "about," and *dies*, meaning "day") **rhythm**. Experiments have been conducted that isolate humans from all external sources of time cues (for example, by having subjects live in bunkers, caves, or a special laboratory environment). In these investigations, the individuals had no idea about sunrise, sunset, light, darkness, time of day, or time for meals. They did not have any clock, telephone, or television. They were allowed to sleep, wake up, and eat whenever they wanted.

Suprachiasmatic nuclei

Cluster of nerve cells within which the human internal clock is thought to reside.

Pituitary gland

The organ responsible for secretion of several important hormones.

Hypothalamus

Center of control for secretion of hormones, food and water intake, body temperature, emotion and sleep-wake regulation.

Retina

The layer of nerve cells at the back of the eye responsible for transmitting visual images to the back of the brain.

Circadian rhythm

The daily pattern of human sleep-wake periods based on the Latin *circa* (about) and *dies* (day).

Under these circumstances (called free running rhythm, because the body's internal clock is not synchronized with the environmental time), the length of the human day appears to be not exactly 24 hours but rather a little longer (close to 25 hours).

When our internal clock is not synchronized with the outside time as shown on a wristwatch or clock, all rhythms (sleep-wake, temperature, and hormone secretion) become desynchronized, which disrupts our normal circadian rhythm. Such disruption is very common in this age of jet travel, when we can quickly cross several time zones. In such a case, the internal body clock does not match with the external clock, which gives time according to sunrise and sunset. This disruption of the circadian rhythm can cause serious sleep disturbances and the undesirable consequences resulting from sleep deprivation (see Questions 6 and 66), including adverse physical effects in our body known as jet lag syndrome (see Question 50).

Although the body can and does resynchronize the internal and external rhythms, this procedure takes time. Indeed, the time required varies depending on the number of time zones crossed, the direction of travel, and the age of the individual. Older individuals tend to take a longer time than younger people to resynchronize the two clocks. In addition, it is more difficult to adjust when traveling to the east than to the west. On average, it takes roughly one hour per day to adjust when traveling to the west, but an hour and a half per day when traveling to the east. Some sleep specialists have suggested that administration of

melatonin, the hormone secreted by the **pineal gland** in the deeper part of the center of the brain at night (which inspired melatonin's nickname, "hormone of darkness"), may help adjust our internal and external clocks. Melatonin does help alleviate jet lag symptoms in some individuals if used appropriately, but it does not help all individuals. Recently, the Food and Drug Administration (FDA) has approved a melatonin receptor agonist drug called Ramelteon (Rozerem™) for treatment of sleep-onset insomnia (see Questions 49 and 53). However, whether this helps patients with jet lag symptoms cannot be answered without further studies.

Melatonin

The hormone secreted by the pineal gland thought to help adjust our internal and external clocks.

Pineal gland

Gland in the center of the brain which secretes melatonin.

The Basics

5. Why do some people go to sleep earlier and others go to sleep later?

Two distinct groups of individuals exist as defined by their sleep habits. Members of one group go to sleep late and wake up late in the morning. These people cannot function well early in the day but become energetic in the evening and function best at that time. These individuals are called evening types (**"owls"**). The members of the other group go to sleep early in the evening and wake up early in the morning. They are energetic and vigorous in the morning but become tired and exhausted in the evening. These individuals are the morning types (**"larks"**). There is also a third group who do not quite fit in the category of morning-ness or evening-ness. A person's sleep habits are probably determined genetically rather than by any environmental factor.

Owls

Group of people, called evening types, who go to sleep late and wake up late in the morning.

Larks

Group of people, called morning types, who go to sleep early in the evening and wake up early in the morning.

6. Why do people sleep at night and not in the daytime? Does a person need to sleep at certain times of the day and night?

Sleep occurs at a particular time during 24 hours. Most of us are used to sleeping at night and waking up during the daytime. Some species (such as rats and bats) sleep during the daytime and are awake during the night; these species are called nocturnal animals.

Humans also need to rest following a period of activity. This rest-activity pattern tends to occur in cycles synchronized with fluctuations of darkness and sunlight and is a fundamental rhythmicity in all living organisms. This rhythm is controlled by both environmental light and darkness and by an intrinsic biological clock, called a **pacemaker**, located in the deeper part of the brain (see Questions 4 and 14). Humans, animals, and plants all follow the basic rest-activity cycle, which is equivalent to the sleep-wakefulness rhythm. The rotation of the earth determines the timing of both the rest-activity cycle and the sleep-wakefulness rhythm.

In addition, the body follows other rhythms, such as the **endocrine rhythm** and temperature regulation. Temperature regulation is most consistently synchronized with the sleep-wake rhythm but follows its own independent rhythm. This fact has been conclusively proven in experiments in which all external time cues (time-givers or **zeitgebers**) were removed, as in time-isolation experiments carried out in the laboratory. Under these circumstances, the body temperature rhythm disso-

Pacemaker

Intrinsic biological clock located in the deeper part of the human brain which controls the rest-activity pattern.

Endocrine rhythm

To come.

Zeitgebers

External time-givers removed during laboratory time-isolation experiments.

ciates from the sleep-wake rhythm and pursues its own independent rhythm.

The body temperature rhythm closely correlates with sleepiness and alertness. At sleep onset at night, body temperature begins to fall. It attains the lowest degree around 3:00 to 4:00 A.M., then begins to rise before final awakening in the early morning. The temperature continues to rise throughout the day, attaining its maximum in the evening. There is, however, a small dip in the temperature in the mid-afternoon. A high temperature favors alertness, whereas a low temperature favors sleepiness. Hence, most humans sleep during the night and remain awake during the daytime, a pattern mainly determined by the circadian rhythm.

Another factor in the human sleep pattern is **homeostasis**, or the maintenance of our internal equilibrium as the body adjusts to physiological processes. Homeostasis ensures that a period of wakefulness is followed by a sleep debt and a propensity to sleep.

Homeostasis

Maintenance of internal equilibrium which ensures that a period of wakefulness is followed by a sleep debt and a propensity to sleep.

7. Why do we dream?

"Dreams: The royal road to the unconscious" so said Sigmund Freud in his seminal book, *The Interpretation of Dreams*, published in 1900. The Freudian theory postulated that repressed feelings are psychologically suppressed or hidden in the unconscious (unaware) mind and often manifested in dreams; sometimes these feelings are expressed as mental disorders or other psychologically determined physical ailments, according to this psychoanalytic theory. In Freud's view, most of the repressed feelings are determined by

The Basics

repressed sexual desires and may appear in dreams as symbols representing sexual organs.

In recent times, Freudian theory has fallen into disrepute. Today, modern scientists try to interpret dreams in anatomical and physiological terms. Nevertheless, we still cannot precisely define "what is dream" and "why we dream."

The field of dream research took a new turn in 1953, when two sleep scientists from the University of Chicago described the dream stage of sleep (or REM sleep) (see Question 1). Approximately 80 percent of our dreams occur in REM sleep and 20 percent occur in NREM sleep. These two states alternate in a cyclical manner four to six times during our nighttime sleep. The last third of the night is dominated by REM sleep. Hence, we dream maximally during late night or in the early hours of the morning.

Although we all dream, we may not always be able to recall these dreams.

Although we all dream, we may not always be able to recall these dreams. It is easier to recall REM dreams than NREM dreams. It is also easier to recall dreams if we are awakened immediately after the onset of REM dreams, rather than trying to remember them the next morning upon getting out of bed. REM dreams are often vivid, unrealistic, and bizarre. In contrast, dream recall, which sometimes may partially occur on awakening immediately from the NREM dream state, is more realistic. Most of our dreams take place in natural color, rather than black and white. In our dreams, we employ all five senses. In general, we use mostly our visual sensations, followed by auditory sensations; tactile, smell, and taste sensations are represented least.

Dreams can be pleasant, unpleasant, frightening, or sad. They generally reflect one's day-to-day activities. Fear, anxiety, and apprehension are incorporated into our dreams. In addition, stressful events of past or present may occupy our dreams. The dream scenes or events are rarely rational but often occur in an irrational manner with rapid change of scene, place, or people (or a bizarre mixture of these elements). Sometimes, lucid dreams may arise in which the dreamer seems to realize vividly that he or she is actually dreaming and may even control the content of dreams.

Some people have frequent, frightening dreams called nightmares or dream anxiety attacks, which appear to arise from intense, anxiety-provoking incidents in the dreamer's life. Nightmares are very common in children, beginning around the age of three to five years. They decrease in old age. Sometimes, during fearful dreams, the individual may enact a past stressful event (for example, a scene in a battlefield or a car accident).

The question of why we dream has both **neurophysiological-neuroanatomical** and psychological interpretations. Sleep scientists try to explain dreams in terms of the anatomical and physiological interpretations of REM (dream stage) sleep. During this stage, the **synapses** (contact points between nerve cells), nerve cells, and nerve fibers connecting various groups of nerve cells in the brain become activated. This activation begins in the **brain stem** (the deeper part in the base of the brain which connects the main brain hemisphere with the spinal cord). The main brain hemisphere then synthesizes these signals and creates colorful or black-and-white images, giving rise to dreams. Similarly, signals sometimes become converted into auditory, tactile, or other sensations to create dream

Neurophysiological-neuroanatomical

One method of interpretation used by sleep scientists to explain the reasons why humans dream.

Synapses

contact points between nerve cells in the brain.

Brain stem

Deeper part in the base of the brain which connects the main brain hemisphere with the spinal cord.

imagery. Why the nerve circuits are stimulated to cause dreaming is not clearly understood. We do know that REM sleep and NREM sleep alternate in a cyclical manner as a result of activation and inhibition of REM-on cells (those activated during REM sleep) and REM-off cells (those remaining quiet during REM sleep).

The main chemical agent causing activation of REM sleep is **acetylcholine**. Several other chemicals (e.g., **noradrenaline, serotonin** and **histamine**) are responsible for inactivation of REM sleep. In addition, the inhibitory neurotransmitter (**gamma-aminobutyric acid-GABA**) plays a very important role in regulating the REM sleep. Thus an imbalance between these brain chemicals may cause nightmares, depression, and some other mental disorders.

Nobel laureate Francis Crick (who discovered the DNA structure) and Graham Mitchison have postulated that during dreams we unburden the brain of useless information. Some have also suggested that memory consolidation takes place during dream stages of sleep. In addition, stories abound regarding artists, writers, and scientists who developed innovative ideas about their art, literature, and scientific projects during dreams.

8. How common are sleep problems?

Day-to-day practice in medicine and various epidemiological surveys undertaken in the United States and elsewhere have made it abundantly clear that sleep problems are very common. Both insomnia and excessive sleepiness are prevalent in our society. In January 1993, a report of the National Commission of Sleep

Acetylcholine

The main chemical agent causing activation of REM sleep.

Noradrenaline

One of the chemicals responsible for inactivation of REM sleep.

Serotonin

One of the chemicals responsible for inactivation of REM sleep.

Histamine

One of the chemicals responsible for inactivation of REM sleep.

Gamma-aminobutyric acid (GABA)

Neurotransmitter that plays an important role in regulating REM as well as NREM sleep.

Both insomnia and excessive sleepiness are prevalent in our society.

Disorders Research stated that millions of Americans are affected by sleep disorders, costing the society billions of dollars. Since the publication of that report, there has been a growing perception of sleep problems amongst the public and professions. Some statistics (see the Introduction) also attest to the seriousness of sleep problems in today's society. In reality, the problems are probably even more prevalent than revealed in these surveys because no standardized definition of insomnia, sleep apnea, or excessive sleepiness exists.

A number of factors are associated with a greater prevalence of sleeplessness or insomnia: old age; female gender; lower socioeconomic status; being divorced, widowed, or separated; depression; stress; drug or alcohol abuse; and certain medical disorders. Sleep deprivation is truly a curse of modern society. In our competitive drive to move ahead in life, we often sacrifice our precious hours of sleep. As a result, we may suffer from excessive daytime sleepiness, which may actually cut our productivity and compromise our safety on the road. Many people do not realize that a sleep-deprived driver is as dangerous as a drunk driver.

Many people do not realize that a sleep-deprived driver is as dangerous as a drunk driver.

Sleep apnea (see Question 39), a very serious condition, remains undiagnosed in thousands of people. Studies performed in Europe, the United States, and Israel clearly show that the prevalence rate for sleep apnea ranged from 1 to 4 percent. Only a handful of such patients are ever referred to a sleep specialist for diagnosis and treatment. Intensive education for both the medical profession and the public is needed to emphasize the existence and seriousness of a variety of disorders affecting our sleep. After all, sleep consumes one-third of our lives.

Sleep apnea

Very serious sleep disturbing condition in which a sleeper stops breathing during the night, resulting in interruptions of the sleep cycle.

9. What are common sleep problems?

Patients with sleep problems most commonly complain of the following:

I cannot sleep.
I cannot stay awake.
I cannot sleep at the right time.
I thrash and move about in bed, and I have repeated leg jerking.

These complaints address the entire field of sleep disturbances. "I cannot sleep" means that the person has trouble falling asleep or staying asleep and wakes up repeatedly throughout the night, including early hours of the morning. "I cannot stay awake" means that he or she falls asleep during the day at inappropriate places and under inappropriate circumstances. "I cannot sleep at the right time" means that the individual experiences difficulty going to sleep at the appropriate time; that is, he or she either goes to sleep late (for example, 3:00 A.M. to 5:00 A.M.) and wakes up late (for example, 11:00 A.M. to 1:00 P.M.), or goes to sleep early (for example, 8:00 P.M. to 9:00 P.M.) and wakes up early (for example, 3:00 A.M. to 5:00 A.M.). The last complaint—thrashing and leg jerking—refers to someone with periodic movements of the legs during sleep at night (witnessed by the bed partner) or thrashing, flailing, and other abnormal movements during sleep. These motions occur in a variety of sleep disorders.

There are more than 80 distinct sleep disorders classified under 8 main categories in the recent International Classification of Sleep Disorders

Insomnia and sleep deprivation are the most common sleep problems in our society today. There are more than 80 distinct sleep disorders classified under 8 main categories in the recent International Classification of Sleep Disorders (Edition 2, 2005, produced by the

American Academy of Sleep Medicine). **Table 1** lists these categories and all of these problems are addressed briefly later in this book.

10. Are sleep disorders serious problems?

Sleep disorders are very serious problems. An occasional night of sleeplessness or daytime sleepiness once in a while is very common and does not need any special consideration. On the other hand, when sleep problems interfere with a person's quality of life and day-to-day function, he or she must consult a physician to avoid serious consequences. Sleep deprivation is pervasive in our society, and the ensuing sleepiness makes us prone to accidents in the workplace and on the road. Indeed, sleep deprivation has been cited as a

Sleep deprivation is pervasive in our society, and the ensuing sleepiness makes us prone to accidents in the workplace and on the road.

Table 1   Common Sleep Problems

- Insomnia (difficulty falling or maintaining sleep, early morning awakening and non-refreshing sleep associated with impairment of daytime functioning)
- Sleep apnea (cessation of breathing during sleep; see Question 39)
- Restless Legs Syndrome (see Question 44) and other related movement disorders
- Narcolepsy (see Question 42) and other causes of excessive daytime sleepiness including behaviorally-induced insufficient sleep syndrome
- Sleep disturbance (insomnia and excessive daytime sleepiness) as a result of general medical, neurological and psychiatric disorders
- Drug- and alcohol-related sleep problems
- Parasomnias (abnormal movements and behaviors occurring during sleep)
- Circadian rhythm sleep disorders (mismatch of timing between the group of nerve cells functioning as a time clock in the center of the brain and the outside clock)

The Basics

major factor in many national and international catastrophes (see the Introduction).

11. Is the sleep pattern different in normal elderly people?

The sleep patterns in normal elderly people do differ from the patterns seen in younger individuals. In particular, the 24-hour sleep-wake schedule is somewhat altered in the elderly. In these individuals, there is phase advance, meaning that the elderly often go to sleep early and wake up early in the morning. Night sleep is considerably decreased, and the total sleep time at night may be decreased. Because older individuals often take daytime naps, however, their total 24-hour sleep time does not appear to differ dramatically from that of young adults.

Elderly individuals often wake up several times during the night, including the early hours of the morning. Their deep dreamless stage of sleep is shorter, whereas the lighter stage of sleep is longer, these physiological changes could reflect age-related changes in the nerve cells controlling the sleep-wake cycles and the circadian rhythm.

12. How does sleep change from birth to old age?

Sleep patterns and sleep requirements change dramatically from newborn to old age in an orderly manner depending on the maturation of the central nervous system. Environmental and genetic factors, as well as any associated illnesses, will have significant effects on such evolutionary changes. Newborns have a **polyphasic sleep pattern** (sleep alternates with waking states on a 3- to 4- hour cycle throughout 24 hours). This is because the biological clock (see Question 4) is not fully developed in the newborn. Sleep occurs at random for a total of about 16 hours a day. About 50% of sleep in the newborn is spent in active sleep (equivalent to REM sleep of adults) and the other half is spent in quiet sleep (NREM sleep of adults). Sleep requirement decreases to about 12 to 14 hours a day between 1 and 3 years of age; by age 5, the average sleep requirement is about 10 hours a day. Napping continues to be about 3 naps a day between 3 and 6 months of age, decreasing to 1 nap a day at age 1 year. Between 4 and 6 years of age, naps are given up. There is progressive change throughout childhood in the form of reduced total sleep time, less napping, reduced slow wave sleep, longer sleep cycles, reduction of arousals, body movements, and rapid eye movements reflecting maturational changes within the brain. In pre-school children, sleep assumes a **biphasic pattern**. Adults exhibit a **monophasic sleep pattern** with consolidated sleep at night with an average duration of 7½ to 8 hours. But this changes back to a biphasic pattern with napping during the daytime in the elderly. The total sleep time in 24 hours in the elderly remains the same, but the night sleep is reduced and this is compensated by taking short naps in the daytime. The exact cause of sleep changes in normal elderly persons is not known but several physiological changes (e.g., decreased melatonin and growth hormone secretion and increased cortisol secretion) may cause alteration

The Basics

Polyphasic sleep pattern

Alternating periods of 3 to 4 hours of sleep and waking observed in newborns.

Biphasic pattern

Sleep pattern observed especially in the elderly wherein napping during the daytime offsets a person's shorter nighttime sleep periods.

Monophasic sleep pattern

Consolidated sleep at night only, as opposed to biphasic sleep pattern of two periods of sleep at night and a short nap in the daytime or polyphasic sleep pattern of several short periods of sleep throughout 24 hours, as in newborn.

of sleep/wake rhythm. As a result of these changes, the elderly take longer to fall asleep and show increased awakenings at night and decreased slow wave sleep.

*Sleep distur-
bance is more
prevalent and
intense in
older people
than it is
in younger
individuals.*

13. What are some sleep problems in old age?

Sleep disturbance is more prevalent and intense in older people than it is in younger individuals. Sleep problems in old age include both normal sleep-related changes (see Question 11) and associated sleep disorders which are listed as follows:

- Insomnia
- Sleep apnea
- Restless Legs Syndrome and Periodic Limb Movements in Sleep
- Sleep disturbances secondary to a variety of general medical disorders (such as lung disease, heart disease, arthritis, and other painful conditions)
- Psychiatric-psychological conditions (such as depression)
- Neurological disorders (such as Parkinson's disease, Alzheimer's disease, and other degenerative diseases of the nervous system)
- Abuse of alcohol, sedative-hypnotic drugs, and other medications
- Rapid eye movement behavior disorder
- Advanced sleep phase syndrome (a disturbance of the circadian rhythm)

The prevalence of sleep apnea increases with age and is greater in men than in women. Insomnia and excessive daytime sleepiness are the two most common complaints in elderly individuals.

A careful history and physical findings followed by appropriate laboratory tests are essential to diagnosing sleep disturbance in the elderly. Many of these conditions are treatable, and treatment can greatly improve the quality of life. In addition to drug treatment, common-sense measures (see Question 56) and participation in regular exercise is important in the treatment of sleep disturbance in the elderly.

14. As we grow older, cells in different body organs, including the brain, progressively decay. If the brain controls sleep, then why is the sleep requirement not decreased in old age?

Some controversy remains about the sleep requirement in old age. Some investigators think that older people need less sleep than younger individuals. Most sleep specialists, however, think that the total 24-hour requirement of sleep in the elderly is the same as that in young persons. Older individuals may wake up repeatedly at night, resulting in a reduction in night sleep, but they often doze off during the daytime, compensating for the loss of sleep at night.

It is true that as we grow older, a progressive decay of cells occurs in different body organs, including the brain. Aging is a biologic maturation process associated with a variety of pathological changes in the central nervous system, including shrinkage and reduction

The Basics

of nerve cells and fibers in the brain. There is loss of some important nerve cells and fibers regulating sleep-wake rhythms in the **brain stem** (that part of the nervous pathway connecting the brain with the spinal cord), the hypothalamus (the group of nerve cells and fibers in the deeper part of the brain that controls both hormone secretion and the sleep-wake rhythm), and the circadian pacemaker (body clock) in the center of the brain. These changes may explain why sleep patterns are different in old age (see Question 11). What determines the exact sleep requirement in humans is not known, but most likely depends on our genetic configuration. A critical mass of nerve cells and fibers is probably required to maintain the sleep-wake rhythm and the sleep requirement. If a marked disturbance of nerve cells and fibers (as may be seen in many diseases of the nervous system) occurs in the areas responsible for sleep-wake regulation, our sleep will be disturbed. The result will be insomnia, excessive sleepiness, or alteration of the timing of sleep.

Brain stem

Deeper part in the base of the brain which connects the main brain hemisphere with the spinal cord.

What determines the exact sleep requirement in humans is not known, but most likely depends on our genetic configuration.

15. Why is it bad to perform physical exercise close to bedtime? Conversely, performing yoga, meditation, or relaxation exercises close to bedtime is conducive to sleep. Why?

Physical exercise tends to increase body metabolism and body temperature, which stimulates the arousal systems (groups of nerve cells and nerve fibers in the deeper part of the brain) and interferes with the onset of sleep. Also, at the onset of sleep, body temperature falls (see Questions 6 and 17); for this reason, exercise-induced rise of body temperature will interfere with sleep. Approximately five to six hours after physical exercise, however, body temperature tends to fall. Consequently, it is good to engage in physical exercise five to six hours before bedtime rather than close to bedtime.

Meditation, yoga, and other relaxation exercises tend to decrease the body metabolism, calm any anxieties or worries, and reduce any external sensory stimulation of the arousal systems. The practice of meditation first became known in ancient India circa 3000 to 4000 B.C. and was brought to the West in the latter part of the last century. It is supposed to control the mind and the body, relaxing the muscles and allaying any existing tension or anxiety. Research into meditation has been limited. Most likely, it helps a person attain a state that precedes the onset of sleep, called **predormitum** (see Question 1). Yoga originated from meditation but focuses on a particular action, such as breathing slowly or deeply or sitting straight in a particular position with the eyes closed and with the mind relaxed. Many other relaxation exercises also help relax the mind and the body. All of these measures are conducive to sleep and have proved beneficial in many patients suffering from chronic insomnia.

Predormitum

A state of diminished perception and control through which a person passes in progressing from wakefulness into the sleep state.

16. Is there a relationship between certain foods and drinks and sleep?

Sleep decreases the motility of the digestive organs. Hence, the digestive system may not be as efficient in sleep as in wakefulness, so the sleeping body may not adequately digest food. For this reason, you should avoid large helpings of spicy foods in the evening before bedtime; otherwise, sleep may be disturbed.

The Basics

In addition, certain foods should be avoided at dinner. Processed foods, which contain chemical additives, may not agree with all individuals. Consumption of an excessive amount of refined carbohydrates (e.g., white flour, sugar, sugar-containing foods such as chocolate, cakes) will put a strain on your stomach by filling up and over-stimulating the digestive system during the process of digestion. Similarly, consumption of high-fat foods will strain the digestive system; you should, there-fore, avoid eating lots of fried foods and cheeses. Some foods may interfere with sleep by over-stimulating the digestive system—for example, raw vegetables, salads, and fruits. These items should be eaten in the daytime, either at lunch or breakfast.

Tryptophan

Serotonin precursor amino acid found in such foods as eggs, fish, bananas, peanuts and hard cheese, which modu-lates sleep.

Other foods are thought to have some sedative actions (e.g., potatoes, pasta, rice). Foods that help produce **tryptophan** may help sleep. Tryptophan, a serotonin precursor, modulates sleep. Foods containing this amino acid include eggs, meat, fish, bananas, peanuts, and hard cheese. Some have suggested that high-carbohydrate-containing foods (bread, rice, pasta) are sleep-inducing, whereas consumption of a high-protein diet promotes alertness. As yet, however, adequate scientific studies have not been conducted to fully support these claims.

Because of its tryptophan content, a glass of milk may promote sleep, although studies of this effect have yielded mixed findings. If you are allergic to milk (i.e., lactose-intolerant), avoid this beverage by all means. Avoid drinking too much liquid in the evening, as it may cause extra trips to the bathroom for urinating in the middle of the night. Avoid tea, coffee, and colas in the evening, as they contain caffeine and act as stimu-lants. In addition, you should avoid consumption of alcohol in the evening.

17. How does a warm bath promote a good night's sleep?

A warm bath raises the body temperature, which gradually falls within the next two to three hours. The falling phase of body temperature is associated with sleep onset. It is, therefore, recommended that you take hot baths roughly two to three hours before bedtime.

Body temperature and sleep-wake rhythms are intimately linked. Body temperature begins to fall at the onset of sleep and reaches its lowest point during the third sleep cycle in the later part of the night. The **hypothalamus** (a group of nerve cells and fibers in the deeper part of the brain) regulates both body temperature and the deep dreamless stage of sleep. If the body temperature increases, the length of this sleep stage increases as well. Conversely, body temperature falls during deep dreamless sleep.

Hypothalamus
Center of control for secretion of hormones, food and water intake, body temperature, emotion and sleep-wake regulation.

18. Does a relationship exist among sleep, the bed and pillows, and environmental light, sound, temperature, and humidity?

A relationship definitely exists among sleep, the bed and pillows, and environmental light, sound, temperature, and humidity. For example, if the bed is too hard or sags in the middle, sleep may be disturbed as a result of muscle aches and pains.

All kinds of pillows, including those made of wood, stone, and ceramic materials, have been described since ancient times in different cultures. Modern pillows are soft and stuffed with feathers, polyester, or foam rubber. People who suffer from allergies should avoid

25

The Basics

Although all kinds of advertisements tout snore-preventing pillows, no rigorous scientific studies have been conducted in a large number of cases to substantiate such claims.

feather-stuffed pillows. Pillows are very personal items, and everyone has his or her favorite. The most important thing is to use a pillow that is comfortable to the neck and head. The neck should not be hyper-extended or hyper-flexed so as to avoid producing neck pain or, in people with disc disease in the neck, to avoid stretching the nerve roots. Instead, the neck should be in a neutral position in a straight line during sleep. Although all kinds of advertisements tout snore-preventing pillows, no rigorous scientific studies have been conducted in a large number of cases to substantiate such claims.

Light and sound are the curse of modern industrial society as far as sleep is concerned. Environmental noise, light, temperature, and humidity may all adversely affect sleep. Sensitivity to noise varies from person to person. Women are more sensitive to noise than men, and elderly people are more noise-sensitive than younger people. At the onset of sleep, environmental noise tends to stimulate our arousal system, making it difficult to fall asleep. Any sudden noise in the middle of the night will awaken most of us from sleep. A stronger noise is needed to awaken a person from the deep stage of sleep (deep dreamless sleep as well as the dreaming stage of sleep) than the lighter stages. Similarly, light and excessive humidity causing sweating will prevent a person from getting to sleep and may awaken him or her in the middle of the night.

To promote sleep, the bedroom should not have excessive noise, light, or humidity. Likewise, the temperature should not be too high or too low. High and low temperatures will affect both the quality and quantity of sleep, causing prolonged sleep latency (time it takes to fall asleep), repeated awakenings, and a reduction of deep dreamless as well as REM sleep.

PART TWO

Risk/ Prevention/ Epidemiology

Insomnia is the most common sleep disorder affecting the general population and is the most common disease encountered in the practice of sleep medicine. Several population surveys have determined that about 35% of the general public has had insomnia complaints and in 10% of the population this is a persistent problem.

Transient insomnia

Also known as short-term or acute insomnia, resulting from an identifiable stressful situation.

19. What causes temporary and long-standing sleeplessness?

Sleeplessness or insomnia may be due to many causes. Sometimes, a given individual may experience more than one cause. Also, different causes may produce different types of insomnia (such as sleep-onset or sleep maintenance insomnia). For example, anxiety may cause sleep-onset problems, whereas depression may lead to early morning insomnia. Insomnia is the most common sleep disorder affecting the general population and is the most common disease encountered in the practice of sleep medicine. Several population surveys have determined that about 35% of the general public has had insomnia complaints and in 10% of the population this is a persistent problem.

Transient and short-term or acute insomnia, also known as adjustment insomnia, is an acute insomnia resulting from an identifiable stressful situation. This generally lasts from a few days to a few weeks and 3 months at most. Once the stressful event is removed and the patient adjusts to the event, the sleep disturbance resolves. The most common cause of acute insomnia is a change in the sleeping environment, for example, sleeping in an unfamiliar environment such as a hotel room, sleep laboratory, or a nursing home or hospital. Unpleasant room temperature, humidity, or excessive environmental noise may also lead to transient insomnia. Acute medical or surgical illnesses and stressful life events (e.g., divorce, stress at work, loss of employment, death of a loved one, preparing for an examination the next day) might also cause transient and short-term insomnia. Some medications (see Question 21) or eating a heavy meal in the evening may cause short-term insomnia. Likewise, taking an airplane flight that crosses several time zones (see

Question 50) may cause transient insomnia. Many of the almost 5 million shift workers in the United States are also prone to short-term or chronic insomnia in addition to other physical problems.

Most cases of insomnia are chronic and **comorbid** (associated with) with other conditions. A variety of psychiatric, medical or neurological illnesses may be associated with chronic insomnia. Other causes include chronic drug and alcohol use. In the past, these comorbid insomnias were classified as secondary insomnia which signifies a cause and effect relationship, but there is no definite evidence that these conditions are responsible for insomnia. Some sleep specialists think that psychological and psychiatric disorders are the most common causes of such long-standing sleep problems. However, many people with insomnia do not have psychiatric or psychological problems. Some common medical disorders associated with insomnia include coronary arterial disease, heart failure, bronchial asthma and chronic obstructive lung disease, peptic ulcer disease, rheumatic disorders, chronic fatigue syndrome, systemic cancer and some skin disorders. Some common neurological conditions associated with insomnia include Parkinson's disease, Alzheimer's disease and other types of dementias, traumatic brain injury, headaches and strokes. In addition, some primary sleep disorders where no cause can be found or associated with insomnia include primary or **psychophysiologic insomnia**. These patients generally suffer from long-standing sleeplessness since childhood. In many of these patients there is a "learned" association between the bedroom and wakefulness. As soon as these patients enter the bedroom and are ready to get to bed, they become anxious which prevents them from relaxation and they become

Comorbid

Pertaining to two or more disorders simultaneously.

Psychophysiologic insomnia

One type of insomnia for which a specific cause cannot be identified.

29

hyperalert. There is some evidence of excessive alertness in some patients as manifested by a variety of physiological changes found in a small group of individuals. Restless Legs Syndrome (see Questions 25, 26, 27, 44, and 45), poor sleep hygiene, and circadian rhythm sleep disorders (see Questions 33, 50 and 51) are some of the other causes of chronic insomnia. Patients who have poor sleep hygiene do not follow any regular sleep/wake schedules and resort to activities which will stimulate the alerting system such as watching television in bed, eating in bed, planning the next day's activities at bedtime, and smoking.

20. Why does pain cause sleeplessness?

Many people have difficulty going to sleep or maintaining sleep throughout the night because of pain. Generally, minor aches and pains do not interfere with sleep. On the other hand, moderate to severe pain (such as cancer pain, pain of arthritis, and neuralgic pain) can very definitely interfere with sleep. Most commonly back pain, followed by headache and other painful conditions, is associated with sleep disturbance.

Pain also includes an emotional component—some patients perceive pain more readily than others do. Emotional factors may stimulate the arousing system (wakefulness system) in the brain, which will have adverse effects on sleep. We need to relax, lie down quietly in bed, and forget about everything else in the wakeful world when we are getting ready to go to sleep. Severe pain may cause physical discomfort, lead to repeated shifting of body position, or make us anxious and tense, thereby stimulating the arousing system and causing frequent awakenings during the night. All of these factors cause both sleep-onset problems and maintenance insomnia.

In addition to its mechanical and psychological effects (such as anxiety and tension), pain may interact with **neurotransmitters** (chemicals responsible for transmitting nerve signals) in the brain. These neurotransmitters (e.g., adrenaline, noradrenaline, serotonin, and acetycholine) have considerable regulatory influence on sleep-wakefulness. For example, a serotonin deficiency in the brain may reduce the threshold for perception of pain, causing us to feel pain very easily and experience sleep disturbance. In a 1996 National Sleep Foundation Gallup survey, about one-third of American adults complained of sleeplessness and nighttime pain, on an average of 8.5 nights a month, sleeping only four hours and 36 minutes during those nights.

Neurotransmitter
Chemical responsible for transmitting nerve signals in the brain.

Another factor that affects sleep in chronic pain sufferers is depression. Many patients with chronic pain suffer from depression, which is an important cause of insomnia in general.

It should be noted that sleep deprivation, particularly REM sleep deprivation may sensitize a patient who is already suffering from pain, causing the pain to be perceived more severely. Thus, REM sleep deprivation may cause **hyperalgesia** (that is, excessive perception of pain) in those already suffering from a painful condition.

Hyperalgesia
Excessive perception of pain.

The treatment for sleep disturbance associated with pain should be directed primarily at alleviation of the pain along with short-term use of sleeping medications. As noted above, it is good to have a good night's sleep rather than sleep deprivation; otherwise there is exacerbation of pain sensitivity resulting from inadequate amount of sleep. This approach is preferred to pre-scribing sleeping medications on a long-term basis.

21. Can medications cause excessive sleepiness or sleeplessness?

Certain medications may cause excessive daytime sleepiness, whereas others may lead to sleeplessness or insomnia.

Many drugs used to treat general medical, neurological and psychiatric illnesses may cause excessive daytime sleepiness and insomnia.

Many drugs used to treat general medical, neurological and psychiatric illnesses may cause excessive daytime sleepiness and insomnia. For instance, antihistamines used to treat allergies and the symptoms of common colds cause daytime sleepiness, as do narcotics (e.g., morphine, codeine) used to treat severe pain. Even aspirin may have a mild hypnotic effect. Likewise, certain medications used to control nausea and vomiting may cause drowsiness. All prescribed and over-the-counter (OTC) sleeping pills, of course, may cause daytime sedation and sleepiness. In addition, many antidepressants and certain drugs used to treat epilepsy may cause daytime sleepiness.

Beta blockers

Class of drugs used to treat high blood pressure and heart disease.

Drugs used to treat high blood pressure and heart disease (e.g., **beta blockers**) may lead to difficulty in sleeping, repeated awakenings during sleep, and night-mares. Nightmares may also be caused by suddenly stopping medications that are REM (dream stage of sleep) suppressants; such agents are often used to treat depression and other psychiatric illnesses. Appetite suppressant drugs are stimulants and, therefore, cause insomnia. In addition, some OTC drugs used to control nasal and sinus congestion are mild stimulants and can lead to difficulty in sleeping.

22. Can certain medications cause excessive dreams?

Certain drugs can increase dreams. For example, L-dopa, pergolide, and other drugs used to treat Parkinson's disease as well as beta blockers and related drugs used to treat high blood pressure can increase dreams and nightmares. Alcohol withdrawal may intensify dreams. In contrast, many antipsychotics and antidepressant medications, as well as some sleeping medications (such as benzodiazepines), may suppress dreams. On withdrawal of these agents, an intensification of dreams and nightmares occurs.

23. Do frequent dreams interfere with sleep?

Frequent, pleasant, or non-frightening dreams generally do not interfere with sleep. Dreamers usually go back to sleep quickly. If the dreams occur daily or several times per week and awaken the dreamer, however, sleep may be disturbed because of exhaustion and failure to go back to sleep rapidly. Individuals who experience nightmares often wake up with sweating, fear, palpitation, and exhaustion. For this reason, frequent nightmares may interfere with sleep.

24. What causes narcolepsy? Can narcolepsy run in the family?

The cause of narcolepsy (see Question 42) was not known to the medical profession until recently. Although the young Austrian neurologist named Von Economo predicted the site of this illness in the beginning of the last century, it was in 1999 that investigators discovered there is a marked reduction of a group of special nerve cells containing a peptide chemical (hypocretin or orexin) located in the hypothalamus (a structure in the deeper part of the brain controlling sleep-wake regulatory mechanisms besides temperature and appetite regulation). However, we still do not know the exact reason why these groups of nerve cells are markedly depleted in these patients. Active research is continuing in this direction and once a cause is found, there will be hope for a medicine to permanently cure the condition.

Narcolepsy can run in the family. Studies have shown that 1 to 2 percent of first-degree relatives of narcoleptic patients present with symptoms of narcolepsy, compared with 0.02 to 0.18 percent of the general population. Studies of twins, however, have shown that this genetic influence is not very strong. Additional environmental factors are important in the causation of narcolepsy.

25. How common is Restless Leg Syndrome (RLS)?

Restless Leg Syndrome (RLS) is a very common neurological and movement disorder but it often remains undiagnosed or under-diagnosed because of misconceptions and lack of knowledge about the entity. The diagnosis is based entirely on the patient's history and physical examination taking into consideration the essential criteria as outlined in Question 44 and there is not a single diagnostic test for RLS. Prevalence (presence of a disease in a segment of population and at a certain point of time) of RLS increases with age. Epidemiological studies have stated the prevalence as varying from 2.5 to 10%. The prevalence of most severe cases (having symptoms at least twice weekly with distress) is approximately 2.5%. These figures are derived mostly from surveys in North American and European populations. In some surveys from Asia, the prevalence is less suggesting a possible ethnic and racial difference in RLS prevalence. Some of the risk factors associated with RLS are increasing age, female gender, pregnancy, iron deficiency, **neuropathy** (affection of peripheral nerves) and end stage kidney disease.

26. Does RLS run in the family?

Family studies of RLS suggest an increased occurrence (about 40-50%) in first-degree relatives of **idiopathic** RLS cases (those not associated with other disease and no causes found). The presence of similar symptoms in such high percentage (40-50%) suggests that RLS follows a dominant mode of inheritance. First- and second-degree relatives of RLS patients are affected more often than are controls. This risk is particularly apparent in patients with an early age of onset (before the age of 45 years). These studies have not yet precisely determined the risk of RLS occurring in close relatives. However, a recent genome-wide association study of RLS identified common variants in certain genomic regions conferring more than 50% increase in risk for RLS.

27. What is the cause of RLS?

Researchers have been trying to identify the cause of RLS since its description more than half a century ago. Today, we know a great deal about RLS—but not exactly what causes RLS or which part of the nervous

*Some of the risk factors associated with RLS are increasing age, female gender, pregnancy, iron deficiency, **neuropathy** (affection of peripheral nerves) and end stage kidney disease.*

Neuropathy
Risk factor for RLS involving affection of peripheral nerves.

Idiopathic
Not associated with other disease and no causes found.

Risk/Prevention/Epidemiology

Brain stem

Deeper part in the base of the brain which connects the main brain hemisphere with the spinal cord.

Spinal Cord

Long tubular structure of the central nervous system that connects to the brain stem and runs through the vertebral column.

Dopamine

Chemical which is deficient in patients with Parkinson's disease.

system, if any, is affected. Is the problem located in the brain, **brain stem** (the lower part of the brain, which is connected to the main portion of brain and controls vital function such as circulation, respiration, and sleep), or the **spinal cord** (the long, tubular structure of the central nervous system that connects to the brain stem and runs through the vertebral column)?

Based on research studies, it appears that the problem lies somewhere between the main portion of the brain (the cerebral hemisphere) and the spinal cord. Response-to-treatment and other studies point to a problem with a chemical called **dopamine**, which is deficient in Parkinson's disease. However, the problem with dopamine in patients with RLS seems to involve a different mechanism than is present in Parkinson's disease. The most current research focus is centered on iron-dopamine dysfunction in RLS. The contemporary thinking in our understanding of RLS suggests an abnormality in the body's use and storage of iron at least in a subgroup of RLS patients. Iron is needed for dopamine synthesis and, therefore, a deficiency of brain iron may contribute to the dopamine dysfunction that is supporting iron-dopamine hypothesis in RLS.

Neurophysiologic and MRI studies suggest that the dysfunction may occur somewhere in the region of the brain stem. In most cases of RLS, no clear cause is found.

In some patients, RLS symptoms may arise secondary to other disorders, such as an abnormality of the nerves conducting impulses outside the central nervous system, chronic failure of the **kidneys** (the organs responsible for urine production and excretion from the body), iron deficiency, diabetes mellitus, or chronic

Kidneys

Organs responsible for urine production and excretion from the body.

joint disease. RLS may also be associated with or caused by some medication (e.g., antidepressants). Because we do not know the exact cause of RLS, we can only treat the symptoms but not cure the disease at present. The good news is that most patients get relief, although they may have to continue taking medication indefinitely.

28. How is RLS treated?

For treating RLS, you must see a physician, preferably a sleep specialist with a special expertise in RLS. The diagnosis first must be established by the physician based on the criteria developed by the International RLS study group (see Question 44) before initiating treatment. Basically, the treatment consists of drug and non-drug treatment. In a very mild case of RLS, non-drug therapy may be the only treatment needed and this measure should also be used in those patients with moderate to severe cases requiring medications. Non-drug treatment includes sleep hygiene measures (see Question 56), avoidance of sleep loss and agents that trigger or aggravate RLS (see **Table 2**). There are anecdotal reports of alternative therapies in RLS such as herbal agents like valerian, various types of essential oils, vibrators, pain relieving ointments such as Ben Gay, and acupuncture. It should be noted that there has not been any scientific study to prove the effectiveness of any of the agents listed.

Drug treatment, which must be prescribed and monitored by the RLS specialist, includes any of the four groups of drugs. **Dopaminergic medication** (agent promoting dopamine function) is the first line of drugs. This agent has been used traditionally to treat

There are anecdotal reports of alternative therapies in RLS such as herbal agents like valerian, various types of essential oils, vibrators, pain relieving ointments such as Ben Gay, and acupuncture. It should be noted that there has not been any scientific study to prove the effectiveness of any of the agents listed.

Dopaminergic medication

Agent promoting dopamine function.

Table 2   Non-Drug Treatment of Restless Legs Syndrome

- General sleep hygiene measures (see Question 56 and Table 8)
- Avoid the following:
  - Caffeine and caffeinated beverages
  - Smoking
  - Alcohol
  - Certain antidepressant medications
  - Antihistamine (most of the over-the-counter sleep medications contain antihistamine)
  - Agents which counteract dopamine (e.g., most medications used to treat psychosis, and anti-nausea medications)
  - Sleep loss
- Mild to moderate exercise
- Physical activity (e.g., leg stretching)
- Massaging the legs before bedtime
- Bath 2-3 hours before bedtime or cold compress (in some patients)
- Remain mentally engaged, e.g., reading

Parkinson's disease and is effective in RLS using a much lower dose than that used to treat Parkinson's disease. Only two of these agents (pramipexole or Mirapex and ropinirole or Requip) are approved by the FDA for treating RLS. Levodopa, although not approved, has been used in RLS, but because of the side effect profile, **dopamine agonists** such as pramipexole or ropinirole are the preferred agents for treating RLS. There are always some individual variations and some patients may respond to one or the other dopamine agonist drug. Your physician should determine this by trial and error. The other drugs which have been used are some anti-epileptic medications (e.g., Gabapentine or Neurontin), Benzodiazepine group of drugs (e.g., Clonazepam or Klonopin and Temazepam or Restoril). In very severe cases of RLS, the opiate group of drugs may have to be used or a combination of drugs may need to be tried. Medica-

Dopamine agonist
Compound that activates dopamine receptors.

tions are generally given 1-2 hours before bedtime. Depending on the timing of symptoms, some patients may require two divided doses, for example, one early in the evening and then another later before bedtime. In severe cases, a daytime dose may be added but symptoms must be differentiated from **augmentation** (see Question 44), which is drug-related exacerbation of symptoms noted mostly with Levodopa but also seen in some cases in other dopamine agonists. Your physician should be able to differentiate augmentation from the severity of the RLS. In many idiopathic RLS patients, serum iron or ferritin (which transports iron) levels may be low and appropriate treatment with iron combined with Vitamin C which promotes iron absorption is recommended.

Augmentation

Characterized by intensification of RLS symptoms, occurring earlier than the initial period and spreading to other parts of the body. It is an adverse effect of dopaminergic medication noted mostly with Levodopa treatment.

29. Can sleep apnea run in the family?

Sleep apnea may sometimes run in the family. In most patients, however, the condition is not familial (see Question 39). Risk factors (factors that may predispose a person to sleep apnea) include hypertension, obesity, alcoholism, and minor abnormalities inside the mouth and face (long uvula, small upper airway space, receding chin). These risk factors may be inherited, which would explain the high occurrence of sleep apnea in some families. There may be genes in the family causing upper airway anatomical abnormalities, abnormal facial features, obesity, and abnormal brain control of breathing which might increase the risk for developing sleep apnea in such families. However, adequate studies to determine familial incidence have not been undertaken.

30. Why does snoring become worse after I drink alcohol?

To understand the answer to this question, you must consider the mechanisms of snoring (see Question 74). Snoring is associated with a reduction of muscle tone in the tongue and other muscles in the throat, which narrows the upper airway space. Alcohol has a direct depressant effect on these muscles, further reducing the muscle tone and allowing the tongue to move back farther, thereby narrowing the upper airway space. As a result of these alcohol-induced changes, the snoring worsens.

31. Why do women have sleep disturbances immediately before and after their menstrual cycles?

The 1998 National Sleep Foundation (NSF) poll found that about 36% of young women reported that their sleep was disturbed two to three nights a month due to discomfort of menstrual cramps and bloating. This was confirmed by the 2007 NSF Sleep in America poll reporting that about 33% of menstruating women say that their sleep is disturbed the week of their cycle. Menstrual sleep problems could take the form of either insomnia or excessive sleepiness. Insomnia usually occurs in the premenstrual period for about one week before menstrual bleeding. Excessive sleepiness occurs around menstrual periods. Sleep difficulty often occurs in the premenstrual phase and continues during the bleeding periods.

Premenstrual Syndrome

Condition, possibly caused by alterations in hormone levels, characterized by several negative symptoms including sleep difficulties similar to those of sleep deprivation.

The **premenstrual syndrome** is characterized by symptoms including depression, anxiety, irritability, difficulty falling asleep, too much sleep, unpleasant dreams, increased awakenings, and excessive tiredness. These symptoms are somewhat similar to those noted after sleep deprivation. Some authors have noted an increase in the amount of sleep and sleep disturbances in the premenstrual phase. In contrast, others have noticed increased awakenings in the premenstrual phase. Thus, the findings to date have been inconsistent.

Sleep problems during the menstrual period may arise because of alterations in levels of the sex hormones (sex steroids). During menstrual bleeding and at the onset of menstruation, both estrogen and progesterone levels fall. In contrast, following ovulation in the middle of the menstrual cycle, levels of these hormones rise. Progesterone affects temperature regulation and causes a slight rise in body temperature. This hormone has a sedative effect.

Some rare individuals have a condition called menstruation-related periodic hypersomnia, which responds to estrogen treatment. Estrogen inhibits progesterone production.

32. Why do pregnant women and women who have just given birth suffer from sleep disturbances?

The 2007 NSF Sleep in America poll reported that most pregnant women (84%) report symptoms of insomnia a few nights each week with 40% also reporting signs of a sleep disorder such as snoring, sleep apnea or Restless Legs Syndrome and 54% of pregnant women report napping at least twice a week. In the same poll, 35% of post-partum women report experiencing

Sleep problems during the menstrual period may arise because of alterations in levels of the sex hormones (sex steroids).

The 2007 NSF Sleep in America poll reported that most pregnant women (84%) report symptoms of insomnia a few nights each week with 40% also reporting signs of a sleep disorder such as snoring, sleep apnea or Restless Legs Syndrome and 54% of pregnant women report napping at least twice a week.

symptoms of a sleep disorder such as snoring, sleep apnea, or RLS. Sleep disturbance during pregnancy and immediately after childbirth may be due to a variety of factors: hormonal imbalance, stress, lower back pain. The exact underlying cause, however, remains unclear.

During pregnancy and for a few weeks after childbirth, repeated awakenings and inadequate amount of sleep may cause daytime tiredness and fatigue. Sleep disturbance during the first trimester of pregnancy includes excessive sleepiness due to hormonal disturbance. In addition, sleep is interrupted because of high frequency of **micturition** at night (resulting from the pressure of the fetus on the pregnant mother's urinary bladder). The sleep problem may somewhat improve in the middle trimester of the pregnancy. Poor sleep, however, is a common complaint in the last trimester. The growing fetus presses on the **diaphragm** (the main muscle of breathing, located at the junction of the chest and abdomen) and urinary bladder, causing some breathing disturbance and frequency of micturition and resulting in sleep disturbances. Other factors causing sleep disruption in the last trimester of pregnancy include lower back pain, fetal movements, heartburn, muscle cramps, and anxiety of impending delivery. Vivid dreams and nightmares may also increase during pregnancy.

Immediately after childbirth, the new mother faces an extra demand as a result of the newborn's irregular feeding and sleep-waking behavior, which causes sleep disruption in the mother. In some cases, depression at this stage may lead to further sleep disturbance.

Micturition

Function of urination, increased frequency of which interferes with sleep.

Diaphragm

Main muscle of breathing, located at the junction of the chest and abdomen.

33. Do night shift workers suffer from physical illness?

Approximately 5 million Americans work during some kind of night or evening shift, and many work on rotating shifts. For example, a person might work during the daytime for one week, then change to night work for the next week, then switch to daytime working hours again. With such a schedule, the internal body clock must readjust frequently. Because of these frequent readjustments, shift workers often suffer from symptoms similar to those of jet lag (see Question 50). Symptoms they may experience include chronic fatigue, sleep disruption, and gastrointestinal symptoms, including peptic ulcer. These problems increase the chance that shift workers will become involved in traffic accidents or make errors on the job. Some researchers believe that shift work can contribute to an increasing risk of heart disease, hypertension, depression and irritability and may pose increased reproductive risks in women such as premature delivery and miscarriage.

Treatment of shift work sleep disorder is challenging and adjusting the work time schedule does not necessarily improve the symptoms experienced by shift workers. Shift workers have disrupted circadian rhythms as they are awake at night and sleeping during the daytime. Treatment should be directed at improving sleep and alertness and realigning circadian rhythms with the sleep-work schedule. In night shift workers, exposure to bright light early during the night shift will be helpful. These workers should avoid exposure to bright morning light on their way home because the bright morning light has an alerting effect and will tend to reset the circadian phase. Hypnotic medications and melatonin have been used during daytime sleep with some benefit. Melatonin, however, is an unapproved agent whose long-term effects are not known. Modafinil, a stimulant medication, has recently been approved by the Food and Drug Administration (FDA) as an agent to help excessive sleepiness in shift work sleep disorders. Modafinil addresses the question of sleepiness but does not address the circadian factor. A sleep specialist should be consulted before using any hypnotic, stimulant or bright light therapy so that the physician can explain the rationale and side effects, and also discuss other social and behavioral factors for optimal treatment of shift work sleep disorders.

34. I have heard that people often have heart attacks, stroke, or even die in their sleep during the early hours of the morning. Is this true and, if so, why?

In an important investigation analyzing the time of sudden cardiac death (related to cessation of heartbeat) in 2203 individuals, a high incidence of death was noted in the early hours of the morning. In a review of the pattern of occurrence of heart attacks and sudden cardiac deaths, another study documented a peak incidence of heart attacks in 11,633 and sudden cardiac deaths in 1981 individuals in the late part of the night and early hours of the morning.

Increased risks of heart attacks, sudden irregular heart rhythm, and stroke have been noted during the late part of the night and early morning when REM sleep (dream stage of sleep) dominates. At those times, blood pressure and heart rate are unstable and there is intermittent activation of the sympathetic division of the **autonomic nervous system** (the part of the nervous system controlling vital functions of the body such as circulation, respiration, and hormone secretion). The amount of blood pumped by the heart decreases during sleep, and particularly during REM sleep in the early morning hours. Oxygen saturation levels in the blood also fall maximally at this time. In addition, adhesion of the **platelets** (special types of blood cells) increases, narrowing the blood vessels to the brain and heart, thereby triggering blood clot formation. All of these factors predispose a person to stroke, heart attacks, sudden irregular heart rhythms, and even sudden cardiac death.

Autonomic nervous system

The part of the nervous system controlling vital functions of the body such as circulation, respiration and hormone secretion.

Platelets

Special types of blood cells involved in clot formation.

PART THREE

Diagnosis

35. How does a sleep specialist diagnose a sleep problem?

A sleep specialist evaluates a sleep problem by first taking a history and then performing a physical examination. Laboratory tests may then be ordered, if necessary.

A sleep specialist evaluates a sleep problem by first taking a history and then performing a physical examination. Laboratory tests may then be ordered, if necessary.

Initially, the physician obtains information regarding the patient's sleep complaints. This history should include not only the problems at sleep onset or during sleep at night, but also symptoms occurring during the daytime. Many patients will complain of difficulty falling asleep, staying asleep, or waking up early in the morning. They may also have excessive sleepiness, irritability, or fatigue during the daytime. Therefore, it is important to have information regarding symptoms during the entire 24-hour period. In addition, the history should cover sleep habits (e.g., bed time, waking time, number of awakenings during sleep at night) and information about drug and alcohol consumption; psychiatric, medical, surgical, and neurological illnesses; history of previous illnesses; and family history. Family history is important because some sleep disorders run in the family, including narcolepsy, RLS, sleep apnea, and sleepwalking.

It is also important to interview the patient's bed partner or caregiver or, in case of children, the parent, to evaluate whether the patient has any abnormal movements, behavior, breathing patterns, or snoring during sleep. The physician should inquire about stress at home, work, or school, as it may cause sleep disturbance.

Sometimes, the sleep specialist will ask the patient to fill out a sleep questionnaire containing a list of questions relating to sleep complaints or ask the patient to maintain a sleep log or diary. This log, which is kept over two weeks, will document bed time, arising time, amount of time needed to fall asleep, nighttime awakenings, total sleep time, mood on arousal and during the daytime, and any daytime naps. The physician may ask some questions to assess subjective evidence of sleepiness. One such tool is the **Epworth Sleepiness Scale**. In this evaluation, the patients rate 8 situations on a scale of 0-3 with 3 indicating a situation in which chances of dozing off are highest. The maximum score is 24 and a score of 10 suggests the presence of excessive sleepiness (see **Table 3**). This scale has been weakly correlated with **multiple sleep latency (MSLT)** scores (see Question 38), which determine objective evidence of sleepiness.

The physical examination is important to uncover any general medical or neurological illnesses, which may cause sleep disorders or be risk factors for sleep dysfunction. After taking a thorough history and completing the physical examination, the sleep specialist will be in a position to suspect the nature of the patient's sleep

Epworth Sleepiness Scale

Tool used during diagnostic process to assess subjective evidence of sleepiness.

Multiple sleep latency (MSLT)

Scoring system used to determine objective evidence of sleepiness.

Diagnosis

Table 3   Epworth Sleepiness Scale

Eight situations	Scores *
1. Sitting and reading	_____
2. Watching television	_____
3. Sitting in a public place (e.g., a theater or a meeting)	_____
4. Sitting in a car as a passenger without a break	_____
5. Lying down to rest in the afternoon	_____
6. Sitting and talking to someone	_____
7. Sitting quietly after lunch without alcohol	_____
8. In a car, while stopped in traffic for a few minutes	_____

*Scale to determine total scores:

0 = Would Never Doze
1 = A Slight Chance of Dozing
2 = Moderate Chance of Dozing
3 = High Chance of Dozing

problem and can order appropriate laboratory tests, if necessary, to confirm the suspected diagnosis. Following confirmation of the diagnosis, the physician will be able to design an appropriate treatment for the problem.

36. What are some important laboratory tests for evaluating sleep problems?

Laboratory tests need to be performed to diagnose some sleep problems. For example, in patients complaining of excessive sleepiness in the daytime, those having difficulty in sleeping at the right time, and those experiencing abnormal movements and behavior frequently during nighttime sleep, laboratory tests are essential to make a definite diagnosis. Such studies are generally not needed in patients with uncomplicated insomnia, but they are necessary if insomnia is associated with periodic limb movements in sleep (see Question 45) or if the patient is suspected of having sleep apnea. Of course, laboratory tests are needed to diagnose the primary condition if the sleep problem is thought to result from a general medical or neurological disorder.

Polysomnographic study

Overnight laboratory test used to diagnose primary sleep problems.

The two most important laboratory tests are overnight **polysomnographic study** (see Question 37) and multiple daytime sleep study (see Question 38). Other tests, which may be needed in special situations, include actigraphy, video-polysomnographic study, and prolonged monitoring of brain wave tests (EEG).

Actigraphy

Test involving wearing a watch-like device on the wrist or ankle to monitor activities of the body resulting from body movements.

Actigraphy involves wearing a watch-like device on the wrist or ankle to monitor activities of the body resulting from body movements—the actigraph is a motion detector. Presumably, we lie relatively immobile during sleep, so the device should register few movements, whereas during wakefulness the actigraph records excessive body movements. In this way, the actigraph indirectly estimates the amount of sleep and wakefulness as well as the time of sleep onset and off-set. The recording is important in patients with circadian rhythm sleep disorders (see Questions 4 and 5), which cause them to experience difficulty in getting to sleep at the right time.

Video-polysomnographic study obtains continuous video monitoring during sleep at night and measures many physiological characteristics (see Question 37) during an overnight study. This test is important to observe any abnormal movements and behavior that may occur during sleep at night so as to make a correct diagnosis. It can differentiate seizures or convulsive movements from other types of abnormal movements and behavior occurring during nighttime sleep. It is important to make a correct diagnosis of each type of movement and behavior in different conditions.

In suspected cases of seizure disorder or epilepsy occurring predominantly at night, it is very important to obtain a prolonged EEG (recording of electrical activity of the brain) both during the daytime and nighttime. In addition, other physiological characteristics during nighttime sleep should be recorded.

37. What is an overnight sleep study? Is it uncomfortable?

An overnight sleep study is a recording of activities from many body systems and organs (physiological characteristics) during sleep at night. It is a painless procedure that should not cause any discomfort to the

Diagnosis

Video-polysomno graphic study
Continuous video monitoring during a sleep study which measures physiological characteristics.

An overnight sleep study is a recording of activities from many body systems and organs (physiological characteristics) during sleep at night. It is a painless procedure that should not cause any discomfort to the patient.

patient. No needles are used, and the subject will not receive any electrical shock. The person having the test is connected by many sensors and wires to the equipment that records various activities. A typical recording continuously registers the electrical activities of the brain (EEG), the muscles (electromyogram, or EMG), eye movements (electro-oculogram, or EOG), heart rhythm (electrocardiogram), respiratory pattern, snoring, body position, and blood oxygen saturation during sleep at night.

Electrical activities of the brain (EEG or electroencephalogram) are recorded by using two to ten channels of a polygraph. The polygraph is somewhat similar to the "lie detector" machine (polygraph test) used in some court cases. Of course, an overnight study takes place in the sleep laboratory, and it records many more physiological characteristics than those studied during lie detector tests.

For EEG recording, electrodes or sensors (small, cup-shaped or flat disks measuring about 5 to 6 mm) are attached with glue to the scalp; these attachments are painless. The sensors are connected by wires to the amplifiers of the polygraph. The electrical activities generated on the surface of the brain are tiny currents that must be augmented or amplified before they can be recognized on the monitor of the computer or recording paper; hence, an amplifier is an essential part of the polygraph. Most laboratories now use computers rather than voluminous amounts of recording paper for recording throughout the night.

To record eye movements (EOG), surface disks are placed over the upper corner of one eye and the lower corner of the other eye. Electrical activities of the muscles (EMG) are routinely recorded by placing sensors over the chin and outer aspects of the upper legs below the knees bilaterally. EEG, EOG, and EMG readings are used to identify the different sleep stages.

In most cases, the respiration pattern is recorded by using three channels. A sensor is placed over the upper lip below the nose to record airflow through the nose and mouth. A band across the chest and another band across the abdomen (strain gauges) register respiratory effort by recording chest and abdominal excursion during breathing. In the most common type of sleep apnea, the airflow channels recording the activities from the sensors placed below the nose show no activity or markedly reduced activity, whereas the channels registering chest and abdominal movements are deflected in opposite directions, indicating obstruction in the upper airway passage in the back of the tongue.

Blood oxygen saturation is recorded throughout the night by using a finger clip. The finger clip registers changes in the color of **hemoglobin** (blood pigment); the color, which is shown on a monitor by a number (for example, 90 to 100 percent in a normal person), indicates blood oxygen saturation (oxygen is carried in the hemoglobin of the blood). In patients with sleep apnea, the oxygen saturation of the blood falls below 90 percent when the breathing (airflow) stops.

Hemoglobin

Blood pigment, the color of which indicates blood oxygen saturation.

To record snoring, a small microphone is attached over the front of the neck. Body position during sleep is monitored through a position sensor over the shoulder. The degree of sleep apnea is worse when a person lies on his or her back. In a routine overnight recording, one channel is used to record electrical signals of the heartbeat (electrocardiogram) via sensors or the electrodes placed over the upper chest.

After placement of all sensors, the connecting wires are gathered into a bundle and attached to the board next to the patient. This board is then connected by wires going through the walls or the ceiling of the bedroom to the main polygraphic machine or computer in an adjacent room, where the technician will monitor a paperless recording (or the paper in the machine, if such a recording is used), and make necessary adjustments to obtain the optimal recording. If any of the electrodes (sensors and detectors) are moved, creating artifacts in the recording, the technician will enter the patient's room and reposition the sensor so that artifacts are eliminated. The technician will also watch the video if such a recording is used (most laboratories generally use simultaneous video recording to observe any abnormal movements and behavior during sleep).

The patient generally comes to the laboratory in the evening around 8:00 P.M. The technician explains the procedure to the patient and tries to set the patient at ease. Making the connections and preparations of the machine and explaining the procedure generally takes one to two hours. The technician then turns the lights off at the approximate bedtime of the particular individual and asks the person to get ready to sleep. If the patient must get up in the middle of the night to visit the bathroom, the bundle of wires can be easily disconnected from the machine and clipped to the patient's pajamas or nightwear, then reconnected again upon returning to bed. In the morning, the technician will come to the room around 6:00 to 7:00 A.M. to turn the lights on, remove the electrodes from the patient's skin, and clean the skin surface. The patient is then ready to go home unless he or she is scheduled to have a multiple daytime sleep study (see Question 38).

38. What is a multiple daytime sleep study?

A multiple daytime sleep study, also known as a **multiple sleep latency test (MSLT)**, is a very important test to assess the severity of daytime sleepiness. MSLT is an absolute necessity for the diagnosis of **narcolepsy** (see Question 42) but is also important to assess the overall severity of sleep apnea and other conditions associated with excessive daytime sleepiness. This test is performed the day after completion of an overnight sleep study. To correctly interpret the significance of the findings in the MSLT, the sleep pattern (total number of hours of sleep and number of awakenings) and the quality of sleep the night before the test must be known. Any impaired and fragmented sleep during the previous night may cause short sleep latency (time to fall asleep) and the appearance of rapid eye movements at sleep onset, thereby introducing confounding factors to the diagnosis of narcolepsy and other disorders causing excessive daytime sleepiness.

MSLT is performed every two hours for four to five recordings, and each recording lasts as long as 20 minutes. The test is conducted two to three hours after the final wake-up in the morning following the all-night study. For example, the test can be performed at 9:00 A.M., 11:00 A.M., 1:00 P.M., and 3:00 P.M. The electrical activities of the brain (EEG), chin muscles (EMG), and eye movements (EOG) are recorded during the 20-minute test. The electrodes for these recordings would have been in place from the overnight study. Patients are asked to refrain from drinking

Multiple sleep latency (MSLT)

Test used to assess the severity of daytime sleepiness.

Narcolepsy

A disorder of excessive sleepiness characterized by a marked reduction of a group of special nerve cells containing certain peptide chemicals.

coffee and smoking in the morning. Following break-fast and explanation of the test, the technician turns the lights off and asks the patient to lie down and try to go to sleep. In between the tests, the patient must stay awake and read, walk around, or watch television but must not fall asleep; otherwise, the significance of the findings will be questionable.

The sleep specialist looks for two findings in the MSLT:

Sleep latency

Time elapsed between lights off and the first onset of any stage of sleep as determined by the changes in brain wave activity.

- **Sleep latency**, which is the time it takes the patient to fall asleep (as determined by the changes in brain wave activity) after the lights are turned off.
- The presence of sleep onset rapid eye movements (the onset of the dream stage of sleep within 15 minutes of the onset of sleep).

Mean sleep latency is then calculated from the values obtained in each nap study. Narcolepsy is strongly suspected if the mean sleep latency is 8 minutes or less (indicating excessive sleepiness) and at least 2 sleep onset rapid eye movements occur in 4 or 5 recordings. In sleep apnea, the mean sleep latency may be 8 minutes or less indicating excessive sleepiness but less than 2 sleep onset rapid eye movements are observed in 4 or 5 nap studies. Any sleep latency of 8 minutes or less is considered excessive sleepiness (pathologic sleepiness). A mean sleep latency between 8 and 10 minutes indicates mild sleepiness and one exceeding 10 minutes is considered normal sleep latency.

39. What is sleep apnea?

The word "apnea" is derived from a Greek word meaning "for want of breath." Apnea—that is, cessation of breathing—occurring during sleep is called **sleep apnea**. Most people, especially after the age of 50 to 60, stop breathing momentarily a few times during nighttime sleep. This condition is normal and not a cause for concern. In a normal person, this breathing cessation may occur as many as five times per hour of sleep. To be significant, the breathing must stop at least 10 seconds during sleep. Sometimes breathing may not stop completely but rather be reduced by 30%–50% of the normal breathing volume, a condition known as **hypopnea**. Like sleep apnea, hypopnea has both short- and long-term adverse effects.

The medical profession has described three types of apneas—obstructive, central, and mixed types. The most common (and most serious) type is obstructive sleep apnea. In this type of abnormal breathing during sleep, the passage of inhaled air becomes obstructed in the region of the upper airway, most commonly at the level of the soft palate (see Question 74). Consequently, air does not enter the lungs (the breathing organs responsible for maintaining normal respiration and blood oxygen at an optimal level), and the blood oxygen level tends to fall below the normal level. The **diaphragm** (the main muscle of breathing, separating the lower chest from the upper abdomen) and other chest wall muscles keep contracting, trying to overcome this obstruction in the upper airway. The brain then sends impulses, telling the subject to wake up. The person then wakes up with a loud snore. As soon as the individual wakes up, the muscle tone in the upper airway and the tongue returns to normal level. The tongue moves forward, the obstruction is relieved, and normal breathing resumes. This cycle repeats as soon as the individual returns to sleep.

Diagnosis

Sleep apnea

Very serious sleep disturbing condition in which a sleeper stops breathing for at least 10 seconds several times during the night, resulting in interruptions of the sleep cycle.

Hypopnea

Reduction of breathing volume to below the normal level.

The medical profession has described three types of apneas— obstructive, central, and mixed types. The most common (and most serious) type is obstructive sleep apnea.

Diaphragm

Main muscle of breathing, located at the junction of the chest and abdomen.

In a mild case of obstructive sleep apnea, the cycle of apnea and normal breathing occurs only a few times. In severe cases, the cycle may repeat several hundred times, repeatedly reducing the blood oxygen level throughout the night and disturbing the individual's sleep. Because he or she obtains an inadequate amount of sleep, the person is sleep-deprived and sleeps excessively in the daytime in an inappropriate place and under inappropriate circumstances.

In central apnea, the airflow stops at the nose and mouth and the air does not enter the lungs. At the same time, the breathing effort by the diaphragm and other muscles of breathing stops. Central apnea is associated with a number of neurological disorders.

Mixed apnea is characterized by an initial period of central apnea, followed by a period of obstructive apnea. In the most common type of upper airway obstructive sleep apnea syndrome, the patient experiences many periods of mixed apneas as well as some central apneas.

Sleep apnea is more common in men than women, although its prevalence increases in postmenopausal women. The male hormone, testosterone, appears to predispose men to sleep apnea, whereas the female hormone, estrogen, acts as a deterrent to sleep apnea.

Researchers have not yet elucidated why the muscle tone in the upper airway falls excessively in patients with sleep apnea, producing an obstruction in the upper airway. In many patients, the **uvula** and soft palate are bulky and long, narrowing the airway passage. In children, large tonsils and **adenoids** (lymphoid tissues in the throat behind the nasal passage) narrow

Sleep apnea is more common in men than women, although its prevalence increases in post–menopausal women.

Uvula

The small piece of soft pear-shaped structure that can be seen dangling down from the soft palate over the back of the tongue.

Adenoids

Lymphoid tissues in the throat behind the nasal passage.

the air passage, causing loud snoring and sleep apnea. The nerve cells responsible for maintaining muscle tone in the tongue and other upper airway muscles appear to transmit fewer impulses to these tissues. To date, no evidence suggests that most patients with sleep apnea have a structural defect in the nerve cells of the brain stem (the lower part of the brain). Of course, neurological disorders (for example, stroke, tumor, trauma, multiple sclerosis) that affect the brain stem or brain may cause sleep apnea in many patients.

Patients with sleep apnea present with a long history of loud snoring, stop breathing repeatedly during sleep at night (witnessed by a bed partner), and are plagued by recurrent awakenings. The major daytime symptom is excessive sleepiness at inappropriate times and under inappropriate circumstances, causing accidents and near-accidents during driving. In long-standing cases of severe sleep apnea, patients may be forgetful and men may have impotence. Although most patients are obese and middle-aged or elderly, the condition can also strike thin people and can occur at a younger age. Therefore, close attention should be paid to the important symptoms of loud snoring, repeated cessation of breathing during sleep at night as witnessed by the bed partner and excessive daytime sleepiness for making an adequate diagnosis because effective treatment will prevent the long-term adverse consequences. These long-term adverse consequences include high blood pressure, coronary arterial disease, heart failure, irregular heart rhythm, stroke, heart attacks and impairment of short-term and long-term memory. In the literature, several inconsistent figures have been quoted for the prevalence of sleep apnea; however, one study which is frequently quoted is that performed at the University of Wisconsin School of Medicine. This

Diagnosis

Patients with sleep apnea present with a long history of loud snoring, stop breathing repeatedly during sleep at night (witnessed by a bed partner), and are plagued by recurrent awakenings.

study stated that about 4% of men and 2% of women were estimated to have sleep apnea syndrome which includes not only the sleep recording abnormalities but also the daytime symptoms. In the same study, analyzing the overnight sleep recording, the figures were 24% of men and 9% of women showing at least 5 episodes per hour of apneas and hypopneas.

40. How is narcolepsy diagnosed?

Most important for the diagnosis of narcolepsy is a consultation with a physician who spends time taking a detailed history of the illness and then performing a physical examination. First, the physician evaluates the nature of the patient's symptoms of sleep attacks and daytime sleepiness. After taking a thorough history, the doctor will perform a physical examination to determine whether any physical illnesses may have caused excessive sleepiness. When the physician suspects narcolepsy, he or she orders laboratory tests to confirm the diagnosis before treating the patient.

The two most important laboratory tests for confirmation of diagnosis of narcolepsy are an overnight sleep study (see Question 37) followed by a multiple sleep latency test (see Question 38). In the overnight sleep study, the narcoleptic patient may fall asleep very quickly and his or her dream stage of sleep (REM sleep—see Question 1) may occur earlier than normal. Multiple sleep latency tests, which consist of four to five nap studies, will show that the narcoleptic goes to sleep much faster than normal people and enters REM sleep within the first 15 minutes of sleep onset in two or more nap studies. Taking into consideration the patient's symptoms, these laboratory abnormalities confirm the clinical suspicion of narcolepsy. The test which has been found to be useful in most cases of narcolepsy with cat-

Cataplexy

Momentary loss of muscle tone without loss of consciousness.

aplexy is an observation of low levels of **hypocretin 1** in the **cerebrospinal fluid** (fluid bathing the central nervous system) obtained by a needle inserted between two lower lumbar vertebrae (in the region of the lower back). This can only be performed in a highly specialized laboratory having the facilities for determination of hypocretin 1 which reflects the activities of the specialized cells containing hypocretin, which are found to be markedly decreased in this condition.

Hypocretin 1

Peptide thought to be important in regulating the sleep/wake cycle.

Cerebrospinal fluid

Fluid bathing the central nervous system.

Diagnosis

41. I am a 60-year-old man who falls asleep in the daytime in inappropriate places and under inappropriate circumstances. I have almost been in two car accidents because of this problem. Should I see my primary physician or a sleep specialist?

Symptoms of excessive sleepiness in the daytime, severe enough to nearly cause car accidents, suggest the presence of a serious condition that requires immediate attention. Many older men have such symptoms.

One common cause of such symptoms in an older man is sleep apnea (see Question 39). Many patients with this disorder remain undiagnosed and underdiagnosed. It is important to identify this condition early to prevent long-term adverse consequences. Fortunately, effective treatment is available for most patients suffering from this problem. To ensure that this condition is treated, you should see your primary care physician. He or she may suggest a consultation with a sleep specialist, who is in the best position to evaluate your condition by performing appropriate laboratory tests and suggesting optimal treatment.

Symptoms of excessive sleepiness in the daytime, severe enough to nearly cause car accidents, suggest the presence of a serious condition that requires immediate attention. Many older men have such symptoms.

42. Since adolescence, I have been falling asleep at class, at work, and while driving. My primary care physician told me I may have narcolepsy. What is narcolepsy?

The French physician Gelineau first coined the term **"narcolepsy,"** which is derived from two Greek words: *narcos* (meaning "sleep") and *lepsis* (meaning "sudden occurrence like a seizure"). Narcolepsy is a chronic or long-standing neurological disorder disrupting the normal sleep-wake schedule and causing an irresistible and uncontrollable desire to fall asleep. The most common age of onset is between 15 and 20 years. The prevalence of narcolepsy is estimated to be about 1 in 2,000 population.

In this disorder, the patient falls asleep in inappropriate places and under inappropriate circumstances. For example, he or she may fall asleep while driving, talking, eating, playing, working, listening to lectures, watching movies or television, being in boring or monotonous circumstances, and even during sexual intercourse. The spells are generally brief, lasting from a few minutes to 15 to 30 minutes. Upon awakening, the narcoleptic individual generally feels refreshed. The attacks persist throughout the patient's lifetime, although treatment provides relief to most people. The diagnosis of this condition is often delayed, however, because many patients are labeled as lazy and inattentive or thought to have misused drugs and alcohol.

Filomena comments:

Before I was diagnosed as having narcolepsy, I literally had been living a very dangerous life. Retrospectively, it is hard

Narcolepsy

A disorder of excessive sleepiness characterized by a marked reduction of a group of special nerve cells containing certain peptide chemicals.

to say exactly how long I had been experiencing the symptoms. During my high school years I don't recall it ever being an issue. While in college, my schedule was so erratic that sleeping an entire day or weekend did not seem unusual. It wasn't until I began driving on a regular basis that I realized something was wrong. I could leave work fully alert and within 15 minutes of driving, I was nodding at the wheel. I've come pretty close to hitting a parked car, knocking off a side mirror, crossing over the double lines and going through a red light. There is no feeling like not having control of yourself. It is very disturbing to think that I not only could harm myself but also take away someone else's life.

I had been told I suffered from hypoglycemia (low blood sugar), chronic fatigue syndrome and just plain old laziness. I was instructed to monitor my caloric intake and to exercise on a regular basis. I began having smaller meals throughout the day and going to the gym five days a week for an hour and a half. Even though I followed my physician's instructions, my sleepiness continued and the frequency of falling asleep started to increase. I continued to inform my primary care physician of my concerns over the years. He then recommended that I have a sleep study and referred me to a sleep center, but I think my results may have surprised him. I'm sure he would have leaned toward sleep apnea before narcolepsy. At the sleep center, the specialist reviewed my history and performed a physical examination. The physician then ordered an overnight sleep study (see Question 37) and multiple sleep latency test (see Question 38) to confirm the clinical diagnosis of narcolepsy.

All patients with narcolepsy have sleep attacks and excessive daytime sleepiness. Many also exhibit other symptoms. Approximately 70 percent of narcoleptics have cataplexy (see Question 43). Other symptoms that are present in almost half of all such patients

All patients with narcolepsy have sleep attacks and excessive daytime sleepiness. Many also exhibit other symptoms. Approximately 70 percent of narcoleptics have cataplexy

include sleep paralysis (a feeling that one cannot move the whole body, one side of the body, or one arm or leg at the onset of sleep or when just waking up), vivid hallucinatory and fearful dreams. Two other common symptoms often noted by patients with narcolepsy are night sleep disturbances and automatic behavior. Because of the disturbance of the sleep-wake regulatory mechanisms, patients with narcolepsy cannot maintain a good consolidated sleep and may wake up repeatedly throughout the night disturbing the sleep. This then adds to the burden of already-existing excessive daytime sleepiness. Automatic behavior indicates performance of the same act repeatedly without being aware of it. For example, the individual may be driving to an unfamiliar place after missing a street sign as a result of brief periods of sleepiness interfering with the attention. Three other sleep disorders are also found to be more commonly occurring in patients with narcolepsy and these include sleep apnea (see Question 39), periodic limb movements in sleep (see Question 45), and rapid eye movement behavior disorder (see Question 46),

43. I suffer from irresistible sleep attacks. Also, on hearing a joke, I tend to go limp momentarily without loss of consciousness. My doctor told me I may have cataplexy. What is cataplexy?

Cataplexy

Momentary loss of muscle tone without loss of consciousness.

Cataplexy is a momentary loss of muscle tone without loss of consciousness, causing a person to fall to the ground; sometimes, just the head may fall forward due to the loss of neck muscle tone or the person may just drop things from the hands. Cataplexy is generally triggered by an emotionally exciting event, such as laughter after hearing a joke, fear, or anger. During these episodes, the patients never lose consciousness. However, sometimes these spells are mistakenly diagnosed as seizures but these are not seizures because there is no loss of consciousness and no other manifestations of seizures such as confusion upon recovering from the spells, injury to the limbs, tongue biting or urinary incontinence. The symptoms of cataplexy make the diagnosis of narcolepsy almost certain, but it is not present in all patients with narcolepsy. Furthermore, in some narcolepsy patients the description of the cataplectic episode is questionable. Generally, sleep attacks and sleepiness occur early during the course of the illness and cataplexy occurs later during narcolepsy in about 70% of the patients—perhaps even months or years later.

44. I am a 65-year-old man. I have terrible feelings in my legs when I am in bed preparing to go to sleep. I must keep moving my legs or get out of bed and walk around to get relief. This condition is driving me crazy and preventing me from getting to sleep. Some doctors told me that it is psychological. Is that true?

The symptoms described here strongly suggest that you may have **restless legs syndrome** (RLS). Karl Ekbom, a Swedish physician, first named and gave a comprehensive description of this disease in 1944–1945. A search of the literature revealed that similar symptoms were described in patients more than 300 years ago by an English physician, Thomas Willis, although he did not name this disease.

Restless Legs Syndrome (RLS)

Common neurological and movement disorder characterized by intense disagreeable sensations and generally prevalent in the evening.

Many misconceptions persist about RLS. Because of a lack of knowledge on the part of many physicians and the public, it remains an undiagnosed or under-diagnosed condition. The symptoms are often thought to be psychological in origin because of their unusual nature. Because of their tendency to occur in the evening or night, physicians do not find any abnormality on physical examination. Restlessness may sometimes be a manifestation of a psychiatric or psychological condition, but this symptom is quite different from the clinical features of a patient suffering from RLS (see below and Questions 25, 26, 27, and 28).

Recently, there has been some bad publicity in the media about the question of RLS. Many individuals who do not have the disease are often skeptical when they hear about this condition or when they see an advertisement on television showing some strange movements of the legs. It has even been suggested that RLS does not exist and that it was invented by the greedy pharmaceutical companies who invest in "disease mongering." This has been a disservice to RLS patients. One just has to ask a patient who suffers from this condition whether this is real or not. Furthermore, recent research linked certain genes to RLS suggesting a biological basis and not an imaginary "disease mongering" condition. Listen to Charlotte's comments:

In June 1983, I was awakened with what felt like a strong electrical shock coming down from the inside of my right knee and shooting down to my ankle. These shocks caused excruciating pain. When I jumped out of bed and stood up, they stopped. I went back to bed, fell asleep for about an hour or two and again was awakened by the same horrible sensations. In the morning, I noticed a large black and blue mark along the inside of my knee which was swollen. I went to the

Emergency Room and was told by the physician that I had burst a blood vessel and to rest. The following two nights, the symptoms returned. On the fourth night, surviving on less than one hour of sleep, my left leg was similarly affected. Throughout the night, each of my legs took turns waking me up after no more than one hour of sleep. My nighttime agony and lack of sleep was affecting my performance at work. It adversely affected my entire life. The quality of my life was worsened. I was constantly exhausted. On the one hand, I could not wait to get into bed and then again I was frightened to do so. I knew the symptoms would reappear as soon as I fell asleep. I lived through years of agony and frustration. I was misdiagnosed constantly. I went from pain clinic to acupuncturists, vascular specialists, internists, neurologists, massage therapists, and underwent epidurals and surgery (for what one physician called a blocked nerve in my leg). I was desperate. The biggest blow I encountered was when I was referred to a psychiatrist who thought all my symptoms were related to my mother's death 43 years ago.

After more than a decade of suffering, I read about RLS in a Canadian medical journal. Finally, I recognized my condition and the realization that all my seven siblings suffered from the same syndrome. I was fortunate enough to find a physician who specialized in RLS and thanks to his empathy and knowledge, I am doing better. Presently, I am the Manhattan support group leader for the Restless Legs Syndrome Foundation, a non-profit organization that aims to empower people and physicians with the basic knowledge of RLS.

Charlotte's description includes the classic symptoms of RLS (see below) and how the symptoms are misdiagnosed for years.

To receive a definitive diagnosis, a patient with the symptoms described in this question should see a physician with a special interest in sleep disorders, especially in RLS. The office of the Restless Legs Syndrome Foundation (see Resources at the end of the book) can direct you to a physician in your area. Several medications can bring relief from RLS symptoms, so it is important to sort things out.

A few years ago, a group of physicians (including the author of this book) who had a special interest in RLS began an effort to develop some minimal clinical criteria for making a diagnosis of RLS. Currently, no single laboratory test can definitively confirm this diagnosis. Likewise, no blood test, nerve test, brain wave test, or X-ray examination of the brain (including the MRI) is capable of proving the presence of this condition. For designing good epidemiological studies for RLS and to standardize the definition and criteria of the diagnosis of RLS for research purposes, in 1995 the International RLS study group published four essential criteria for the diagnosis of RLS which were slightly modified in 2003. These essential criteria are summarized in **Table 4**:

Table 4   Four Essential Criteria for the Diagnosis of RLS

Criteria 1:   An urge to move the legs, usually accompanied or caused by uncomfortable sensations in the legs

Criteria 2:   The urge to move, or unpleasant sensations which begin or worsen during periods of rest or inactivity such as lying or sitting

Criteria 3:   The urge to move or unpleasant sensations which are partially or totally relieved by movements such as walking or stretching, at least as long as the activity continues

Criteria 4:   The urge to move or unpleasant sensations which are worse in the evening or night than during the day or which occur only in the evening or at night

---

All four of the essential criteria must be met with or without the supportive and associated features (described below).

Individuals suffering from RLS develop an intense, disagreeable feeling, variously described as creeping, crawling, tingling, burning, aching, cramping, vise-like, itchy, much like bugs crawling under the skin. Most of the patients, particularly in the early stage of the disease, have noted this in the evening while resting in bed. However, in severe cases, movements may be noticed in the daytime when subjects are sitting or lying down.

The uncomfortable sensations occur mostly between the knees and ankles, causing an intense urge to move the legs to relieve these feelings. About 15% to 20% of RLS patients complain of actual pain. Sometimes the patients complain of similar symptoms in the arms or in other parts of the body, particularly in advanced stages of the disease or when the patient develops "augmentation" (this occurs mostly in patients who have been on Levodopa [the original dopaminergic medication to treat Parkinson's and RLS] for a long time) which is really an adverse affect of Levodopa treatment and the patient's symptoms will occur earlier than the initial period with more intense symptoms and spread to other body parts. These symptoms of augmentation will be made worse by increasing the dose of Levodopa, differentiating it from manifestations of severe disease which should respond to increasing the doses of dopaminergic medication. These symptoms have been noted mostly after Levodopa treatment but have also been described in patients on other dopaminergic medications.

Many patients try all types of tricks to obtain relief from their condition. They move, massage, or rub their legs; they get out of bed to walk around. These maneuvers may temporarily relieve the symptoms. For some individuals, a hot bath may prove helpful. In more severe cases, symptoms may even occur in the daytime when patients are sitting or lying down. Long travel in a car, train, or plane may be particularly distressing. Many individuals with RLS find it impossible to sit for any length of time in a movie house or theater; they find that they must stand in the back of the theater to relieve the intense, disagreeable feelings in their legs.

Other criteria developed by the International RLS study group to define RLS include supportive features: Response, at least in the beginning, to dopaminergic medications (see Question 28); abnormal movements of the legs called periodic limb movement in sleep (see Question 45); and familial occurrence (see Question 26) and associated features (sleep disturbance; normal neurological examination in those cases of RLS where it is not associated with other conditions and no cause is found; and usually chronic progressive course). RLS may have a profound impact on sleep and often the patient seeks medical attention because of the inability to obtain a good night's sleep which is generally a problem of falling asleep but also has difficulty maintaining sleep due to the associated leg movements. Indeed sometimes the individual will wake up in the middle of the night with these feelings, which prevent him or her from having a good-quality sleep. RLS may have the greatest impact on sleep compared with other sleep disorders. These sleep problems may affect the quality of life, including impairment of attention and daytime mood. Because of chronic sleep disturbance, lack of energy and inability to think properly in the daytime due to the sleep deprivation, these patients may also suffer from anxiety and depression. Fortunately, many of these patients will improve their quality of life after receiving adequate treatment for RLS.

Most patients with this condition consult a physician when they reach middle age or their later years. On questioning, however, most will report having symptoms since a young age; because the symptoms were milder then, patients often did not bother to see a physician when they first arose. A few cases of RLS have been described in children, and an association between childhood RLS and attention-deficit/hyperactivity disorder has been reported. The course of RLS is generally chronic, but sometimes remission occurs. The condition may be first noted during pregnancy; it can also be exacerbated by pregnancy. Likewise, ingestion of caffeinated beverages may make the symptoms worse.

45. My husband tells me that I keep moving my legs during sleep. In the daytime, I feel tired and irritable. I do not seem to have quality sleep at night. Do I have RLS?

The symptoms described here suggest that you may have **periodic limb movements in sleep (PLMS)**. In PLMS, certain kinds of movements affect mostly the legs but occasionally the arms; these movements occur in a periodic or semi-periodic manner during sleep, mostly during NREM sleep (see Question 1). The patient moves his or her legs in a periodic fashion, for perhaps an hour or so, and then stops moving. The movements recur intermittently throughout the night. During the dream stage of sleep (REM sleep), they generally stop. The bed partner may be able to describe your movements, which usually include bending of the toes and foot upward, sometimes bending of the knees, and occasionally bending of the arms and forearms every 20 to 40 seconds (range of 5 to 90 seconds).

Periodic limb movements in sleep (PLMS)

Disorder characterized by periodic or semi-periodic movements of the limbs, mostly during NREM sleep.

During some of these movements, the patient may briefly wake up. Although the PLMS patient may be unaware of this awakening, a sleep specialist can detect it by looking at the brain waves (EEG) during an overnight polysomnographic study (see Question 37). The brain wakes up briefly (3 to 14 seconds), causing the EEG to show a change from sleep to waking rhythms (see Question 1). If you briefly wake up in this manner repeatedly throughout the night, your sleep will not be consolidated. The resulting poor quality of sleep will lead to daytime fatigue and sleepiness. Whether PLMS causes sleep disturbance, giving rise to daytime fatigue and tiredness, remains somewhat controversial.

At least 80 percent of patients with RLS have PLMS. In addition, PLMS may occasionally occur as an isolated condition or be associated with a variety of other medical and neurological illnesses, medications, or primary sleep disorders. PLMS has been noted in a large percentage of patients with narcolepsy (see Question 42), obstructive sleep apnea syndrome (see Question 39), and rapid eye movement behavior disorder (see Question 46). In particular, some antidepressant medications may aggravate these movements. Sometimes PLMS may occur in normal individuals, particularly elderly subjects. It should be noted that in some patients with RLS, the abnormal leg movements may be noted during wakefulness when these are called periodic limb movements in wakefulness (PLMW) and both PLMS and PLMW can be diagnosed from the recordings during an overnight sleep study (see Question 37).

To ascertain whether the patient has RLS, the physician will first ask several questions to decide whether he or she meets the minimal criteria established by the

International RLS study group (see Table 4) and then perform a thorough physical examination. Based on the history and physical examination, the physician with a special interest in RLS should be able to differentiate RLS from other conditions which may mimic RLS and may be able to determine whether the RLS has any cause or is associated with other conditions (e.g., iron deficiency anemia, pregnancy, kidney disease, etc.). The physician may ask for some laboratory tests to differentiate RLS from these other conditions.

46. My husband, aged 65, is a perfect gentleman in the daytime. Lately, however, he has begun to behave in an obnoxious manner in the middle to late part of the night. He will kick me, thrash about in bed, and scream loudly. Is he developing a dreadful psychiatric illness?

From the history, it does not appear that the husband is developing a psychiatric illness. A psychiatric illness will present with symptoms not just during nighttime, but also during daytime. The symptoms described here are very characteristic of a condition called **rapid eye movement sleep behavior disorder (RBD)**. This dysfunction occurs in middle-aged to elderly people (more often in men) and occurs during the dream stage of sleep (REM sleep). Because the dream stage of sleep is more intense and prolonged in the middle to late part of the night, the symptoms generally appear at that time.

Patients present with dream enactment behavior, suddenly dreaming as if people are chasing them; in response, they attempt to beat or kick the imaginary

Rapid eye movement sleep behavior disorder (RBD)

Dysfunction occurring in middle-aged to elderly people during REM sleep, characterized by dream enactment behavior.

73

assailant. For example, a patient might imagine that a person is chasing him and consequently kick and thrash the bed partner lying next to him. Often, the affected individual will scream and shout, repeating the same things over and over. Sometimes, he or she may have pleasant dreams; most of the time, however, the dreams are fearful and violent in nature. On many occasions, the patient may cause injury to himself or herself as well as to the bed partner.

Taking a careful history of the episodes and particularly the timing of their occurrence at night may direct attention to the possibility of RBD in a particular patient. It is very important to consult a specialist if a suspicion of abnormal behavior in sleep at night arises. RBD can be treated effectively with a small dose of a benzodiazepine (hypnotic medication). The diagnosis must be confirmed by an overnight sleep study, using a simultaneous video recording to correlate the behavior with the sleep stages. In less than half of all RBD patients, no cause is found. In more than 50% of the patients, many causes are implicated, particularly neurological disorders such as Parkinson's disease, diffuse **Lewy Body disease** (a chronic degenerative neurological illness resembling Parkinson's disease with dementia but differing from Parkinson's disease because of fluctuating cognition, recurrent visual hallucinations, that is seeing things that are not present, repeated falls and sensitivity to antipsychotic medications) and **multiple system atrophy** (a chronic degenerative disease of the nervous system associated with features of Parkinson's disease such as stiffness of the muscles, shakiness of the limbs and slowness of the movements and features of the disease affecting the **cerebellum**, [a structure located below the main brain hemisphere which controls movements and coordination] as well as alteration of the function of the

Lewy Body disease
Chronic degenerative neurological illness resembling Parkinson's disease with dementia.

Multiple system atrophy
Chronic degenerative disease of the nervous system associated with features of Parkinson's disease.

Cerebellum
Structure located below the main brain hemisphere which controls movements and coordination.

involuntary nervous system controlling blood pressure, heart and circulation, regulation of breathing, urinary bladder, sweating mechanism and secretions of the stomach and intestines). In addition, alcohol abuse and some antidepressant and antipsychotic medications may cause this type of behavior acutely. The literature includes many reports of RBD that precede the development of neurodegenerative diseases such as Parkinson's disease, diffuse Lewy Body disease with dementia and multiple system atrophy many years later.

47. My 12-year-old daughter falls asleep normally. Approximately 45 to 60 minutes later, she sits up in bed with a vacant and confused appearance. She then stands up in bed and screams loudly. Sometimes, she exhibits thrashing movements of her limbs. Does my daughter suffer from an epileptic seizure or an abnormal sleep disorder?

Two conditions should be considered in this case: a nocturnal epileptic seizure and night terror, an abnormal behavior occurring during the partial awakening stage. Because the two conditions may be difficult to distinguish, you should consult your family physician to seek a referral to a pediatrician or a sleep specialist for appropriate investigation and treatment.

An epileptic seizure generally lasts for a few seconds to a minute or two and is followed by a period of confusion. The episode may begin with the individual having a vacant and confused appearance but is often followed by generalized convulsive movements of the body. The seizure may be associated with loss of control of urine and tongue biting. A nocturnal seizure may occur at any time of the night and in any sleep stage, though it is most commonly observed in the dreamless stages of sleep rather than in the dreaming stage. Often, the patient gives a history of similar seizures during the daytime. In some cases, however, episodes have occurred exclusively during the night.

Night terror is a partial arousal disorder (like sleepwalking) that occurs during the first third of the night. In the medical profession, night terror or sleep terror is also known as pavor nocturnus. Like sleepwalking, night terror is common in children, occurring between the ages of 5 and 7 years. There is a high frequency of occurrence in multiple members of the same family. During the episode, the patient may sit up with a confused and frightened look and, within a short period, scream loudly with a piercing cry. He or she may begin to breathe very heavily and deeply; the patient's pulse rate may also be very rapid. Most of the time, the individual sits up or stands up in bed; sometimes, however, he or she may get out of bed and walk toward the door. The night terror episode generally lasts only a few minutes, and the patient does not recall the event the next morning.

Many affected individuals also have a history of sleepwalking episodes. Indeed, the triggering factors for sleep terror are similar to those for sleepwalking. Sleep terror is less common than sleepwalking.

If the episodes of night terror occur infrequently and a diagnosis of nocturnal seizure has been excluded, then the only treatment required is preventive measures like those described for sleepwalking. If sleep terrors occur repeatedly and if questions about the diagnosis arise,

Night terror

Partial arousal disorder (like sleepwalking); also known as *pavor nocturnus.*

Like sleepwalking, night terror is common in children, occurring between the ages of 5 and 7 years. There is a high frequency of occurrence in multiple members of the same family.

an overnight sleep study should be performed using a simultaneous video recording and multiple channels to record brain wave activities. Also, psychotherapy and stress reduction measures may be prescribed, and the patient may be administered small doses of a benzodiazepine or a tricyclic antidepressant. If nocturnal seizure disorder is strongly suspected, then in addition to the simultaneous video recording during overnight sleep study, prolonged recordings of brain wave activities may be needed during the daytime.

The other condition that should be considered in such cases is **nightmare**, which is also known as dream anxiety attack. These vivid and frightening dreams, which are mostly visual but sometimes auditory, occur during the dream stage of sleep. That is, they arise during the middle to late part of the night, when REM sleep is more intense and prolonged. Nightmares are very common. In fact, at least 50 percent of all children experience nightmares, beginning at ages 3 to 5 years. Nightmares are generally not associated with motor activities or a state of confusion. A person experiencing a nightmare may recall part of the dream the next morning.

Nightmare
Vivid and frightening dreams, also known as dream anxiety attack.

Nightmares are very common. In fact, at least 50 percent of all children experience nightmares, beginning at ages 3 to 5 years.

48. I am a 40-year-old single woman. I can fall asleep easily but wake up between 3:00 and 4:00 A.M. and cannot get back to sleep again. What should I do?

Early morning awakening is a very common sleep-related problem. Before anything can be done about it, it is important to try to find out why the patient wakes up late at night or in the early hours of the morning. This type of sleeplessness is a symptom, rather than a disease.

A common cause for such a problem is depression. The individual and his or her physician must find out whether symptoms of depression are present. Do you feel sad? Do you feel lonely? Do you feel like sitting and doing nothing? Do you suffer from a lack of energy? Do you feel exhausted and tired all the time? Did something happen at home or in the workplace, which may have made you feel depressed?

Another cause of early morning awakening is drinking alcohol at bedtime. Many people drink alcohol to get to sleep. Alcohol acts as a depressant to the central nervous system. When the blood alcohol level falls, however, rebound awakening occurs; it causes you to wake up early in the morning.

Other causes of early morning awakening may include intense fearful dreams or nightmares, waning of the effects of a sleeping medication taken earlier in the evening, and dependence on sleeping medications. If you cannot explain your problem or think you may suffer from depression, consult a physician. Such problems are treatable and you may not actually suffer from sleeplessness.

49. I toss and turn in bed and it takes me two to three hours to go to sleep. In the daytime, I feel irritable and tired. What is happening to me?

Sleep onset insomnia

Sleep disorder in which the patient is unable to fall asleep for long periods, resulting in insufficient rest and daytime tiredness.

In this case, the culprit is **sleep-onset insomnia**. An estimated one-third of the population suffers from some form of insomnia (either sleep-onset or sleep maintenance insomnia with repeated awakenings). In

10 percent of all people, this condition is a persistent problem (see Question 19). If you do not receive adequate hours of sleep, you will not have quality sleep and will suffer from next day consequences such as irritability, tiredness, lack of concentration and daytime sleepiness(see Question 53 for evaluaion and treatment).

50. Why do I feel bad for days after flying from New York City to Hong Kong and then back to New York City? Can anything be done to help me?

In these days of increasing jet travel that crosses several time zones (for business or pleasure), certain undesirable symptoms that constitute **jet lag syndrome** are commonplace. The result of such travel is that the body's internal clock becomes out of synch with the external clock in the new time zone(see Question 4). When the body wants to sleep, the external environment in the new time zone reminds you to stay awake. This desynchronization causes tiredness, sleepiness, general malaise, impairment of judgment and concentration, and sometimes disorientation. These symptoms, which result primarily from sleep disruption, may also be associated with gastrointestinal problems. The body's other rhythms—including those that control endocrine secretions, body temperature, and gastrointestinal motility and secretions—are affected by crossing time zones. These symptoms may last for several days, depending on the direction of travel and the number of time zones traversed. They also depend on age—older individuals take a longer time to readjust than younger individuals.

An estimated one-third of the population suffers from some form of insomnia (either sleep-onset or sleep maintenance insomnia with repeated awakenings). In 10 percent of all people, this condition is a persistent problem

Diagnosis

Jet lag syndrome

Condition caused by travel outside one's own time zone in which the body's internal clock becomes out of synch with the external clock in a new time zone.

It takes longer to resynchronize the internal and external clocks when traveling east than when traveling west. In general, it takes approximately one and a half hours per day to readjust the internal body clock when traveling east as compared with one hour per day when traveling west. Because our body rhythm does not last exactly 24 hours (it is roughly 25 hours), it is easier to lengthen a day (for example, when traveling in a westerly direction) than to shorten a day (for example, when traveling east). When you are traveling east, your internal body clock lags behind the new local time. For example, at midnight local time in Hong Kong, the body clock in New York City will be noon; consequently, if you travel from New York to Hong Kong, you will not be ready to go to sleep at midnight in Hong Kong. After staying one to two weeks in Hong Kong on vacation or business, however, your body clock will become adjusted to Hong Kong time. Then, when you return to New York, your body clock will remain on Hong Kong time. For example, at 11:00 P.M. Hong Kong time you will be ready to go to sleep, but the local clock in New York City will read 11:00 A.M. so you must force yourself to stay awake.

In addition to the problem of disruption of synchronization between the body's inner clock and its external time cues, other factors contribute to jet lag syndrome: limited mobility while flying, dryness of the eyes on the plane, headache, fatigue, gastrointestinal disturbances, and nasal congestion.

You can take several steps to minimize jet lag symptoms. You should adjust your sleep schedule to the local time on arrival, trying to stay awake during the local daytime. If you can adjust to the destination time for a few days before travel, it will help. Unfortunately, from a practical point of view, this step is rarely possible. Avoid consuming alcohol on the airplane flight; at high altitudes, effects of alcohol may be accentuated, causing sleep disturbance. Taking a sleeping pill at night during a long flight may help. You should never mix sleeping pills with alcohol, however, as this combination may prove lethal.

Exposure to light at an appropriate time might help, though the timing of the light-darkness is critical. For instance, exposure to daylight in the morning of the local time for a few hours while traveling east—to advance the internal clock—may help relieve jet lag symptoms. In the evening of the local eastern time, avoid bright light exposure (wear sunglasses or goggles). These steps should be reversed when traveling west. When traveling east, you advance your body clock; when traveling west, you delay it. It may be advisable to take a short-acting sleeping pill for the first two nights on arriving at the new destination, and after a few days you should overcome your jet lag symptoms.

The role of melatonin for the treatment of jet lag symptoms remains controversial. Some advise taking 3 to 5 mg of melatonin two days before travel at bedtime of the new time zone, with treatment at bedtime continuing in the new time zone for three days. This schedule should be reversed when returning to the original time zone. In general, treatment of jet lag syndrome remains unsatisfactory.

Taking a sleeping pill at night during a long flight may help. You should never mix sleeping pills with alcohol, however, as this combination may prove lethal.

Diagnosis

51. All my life, I have experienced difficulty getting to sleep. I go to sleep between 3:00 and 5:00 A.M. and wake up between 10:00 A.M. and 1:00 P.M. If I have to wake up early, I cannot function adequately. Why is my sleep pattern different from that of the average person?

Delayed sleep phase syndrome (DSPS) is a condition in which the major sleep episode is delayed relative to the desired clock time. This delay makes it difficult to fall asleep and to wake up at the desired time. Patients with this problem have great difficulty in functioning properly during daytime hours, if they must awake early to go to work or school. Because of their disturbed sleep schedules, they cannot function normally in society.

Delayed sleep phase syndrome (DSPS)

Condition in which the major sleep episode is delayed relative to the desired clock time.

The onset of DSPS generally occurs during childhood or adolescence. The condition results from an abnormality in the biological clock located in the deeper part of the brain (see Question 4). Some patients may also suffer from depression.

This type of sleep schedule problem can be clearly documented by keeping a sleep log for one to two weeks and by recording sleep-wake activities with an **actigraph** (a watch-like device that you wear on your wrist for several days; the computer chips in the device record the data that can be downloaded into a personal computer). Several lines of treatment exist, including delaying sleep onset by two to three hours every day until the desired bedtime has been achieved. In addition, exposure to bright light in the morning, some-

Actigraphy

Test involving wearing a watch-like device on the wrist or ankle to monitor activities of the body resulting from body movements.

times in combination with melatonin at night may be helpful. A sleep specialist can determine the best choice of therapy for your case.

52. Is sudden infant death syndrome (crib death) a special type of sleep-related breathing disorder?

A National Institutes of Health panel defines **sudden infant death syndrome (SIDS**; also known as crib death) as the sudden death of an infant younger than one year of age, for which no cause is found after a careful review of the history, an investigation of the death scene, and a complete postmortem examination. The exact cause of SIDS remains unknown. The peak age for such events is between 2 and 4 months, with a range from 1 to 12 months.

Sleep-related breathing disorder is just one suggested cause of this syndrome. The apnea (cessation of breathing) hypothesis for SIDS was first suggested in the 1970s based on the fact that some SIDS victims had a history of life-threatening apnea. After many years of investigation, however, no clear relationship between a breathing disorder and SIDS has emerged.

Epidemiological studies have suggested some risk factors for SIDS: young age of the mother, multiple pregnancies, multiple births, low socioeconomic status, male sex of the baby, low birth weight of the newborn, poor prenatal care, anemia in the mother, and use of tobacco by the mother. Most SIDS victims do not have such risk factors, however, and few have a prior history of apnea. An important factor may be immaturity of the nervous system—particularly those nerve

Sudden infant death syndrome (SIDS)

Also known as crib death, the sudden death of an infant younger than one year of age, for which no cause is found.

cells and fibers that are responsible for the sleep-wake-fulness cycle and the systems responsible for arousing the brain.

Infant-parent co-sleeping has been speculated to reduce the risk of SIDS. Hazards of substance and alcohol abuse by the parents must be considered when advocating co-sleeping, however.

An important consideration that has emerged recently is the danger of accidental suffocation when the infant is sleeping in the prone position. The American Academy of Pediatrics has recommended that infants be positioned on their side or on their back during sleep. Since these recommendations have been widely publicized, the incidence of SIDS has decreased considerably. Unfortunately, many mothers remain unaware of them and do not follow these life-saving guidelines. Recent research has uncovered an abnormality of serotonin (a chemical in the brain) showing decreased binding of receptors in the nerve cells containing serotonin in the region of the **medulla** (part of the brain below the brain hemisphere controlling vital functions such as regulation of respiration, heart and circulation). This chemical abnormality is thought to be developmental in origin. Combined with the various risk factors described above, this brain abnormality may trigger the occurrence of SIDS. However, further studies are needed to understand the implication of this finding, particularly in terms of treatment.

Medulla

Part of the brain below the brain hemisphere controlling vital functions such as respiration, heart and circulation.

PART FOUR

Treatment

53. What can I do for my sleeplessness?

If your problem is more than just an occasional occurrence and interferes with the quality of your life at home and work, you must seek help. First, you may try some common-sense measures to improve your sleep (see Question 56). If the problem persists, you must consult a physician (preferably a sleep specialist), who is in the best position to determine the cause of your sleeplessness after obtaining a detailed history and performing a physical examination. In most cases, the findings will be that insomnia is not a disease but rather a symptom.

In most cases, the findings will be that insomnia is not a disease but rather a symptom.

The specialist will advise you about appropriate treatment, which could consist of sleeping medications or non-drug treatment, or a combination of the two measures. Sleeping medications are generally prescribed for transient and short-term insomnia. In contrast, non-drug treatment, with or without intermittent use of sleeping medications, is the mainstay of treatment for chronic insomnia.

A variety of hypnotic medications have been used to treat insomnia over the years but only a few of them have been approved by the Food and Drug Administration (FDA).

A variety of hypnotic medications have been used to treat insomnia over the years but only a few of them have been approved by the Food and Drug Administration (FDA). Most of these approved drugs act through gamma-aminobutyric acid (GABA) receptor complex. **GABA** is a chemical substance that causes inhibition of activity of the nerve cells and fibers in many sites in the central nervous system. Two classes of such medications have been approved by the FDA for treating insomnia (particularly acute or transient and short-term insomnia): Benzodiazepine receptor agonists and non-Benzodiazepine receptor agonists (Table 5). Since the availability of non-Benzodiazepine receptor agonists during the last several years, these drugs have

Gamma-amino-butyric acid (GABA)

Neurotransmitter that plays an important role in regulating REM as well as NREM sleep.

been used in preference to Benzodiazepine receptor agonists because side effects, and particularly day-after hangover effects, are fewer. Two of the non-Benzodiazepine receptor drugs, Eszopiclone (Lunesta) and Zolpidem-CR (Ambien-CR), have been found in double-blind, placebo-controlled clinical trials to be relatively safe for use up to 6 months. The FDA also approved the use of the first non-Benzodiazepine receptor agonist hypnotic for use in patients with sleep-onset insomnia. This drug, Ramelteon (Rozerem), is a melatonin receptor agonist promoting sleep induction (see **Table 5**). When taking sleeping medications, you must be prepared to go to bed immediately after taking the medication and prepare to have a full night's sleep without getting up and engaging in other activities after taking the sleeping medication. If you do not

When taking sleeping medications, you must be prepared to go to bed immediately after taking the medication and prepare to have a full night's sleep without getting up and engaging in other activities after taking the sleeping medication.

Table 5   FDA-Approved Benzodiazepine and Melatonin Receptor Agonists Indicated for the Treatment of Insomnia

Benzodiazepine receptor agonists: Benzodiazepines

- Triazolam (Halcion): very short acting with half-life of 1.5 to 5.5 hours
- Temazepam (Restoril): short acting with a half-life of 6 to 16 hours
- Estazolam (Prosom): intermediate acting with a half-life of 10 to 24 hours
- Flurazepam (Dalmane): long acting with a half-life of 47 to 100 hours
- Quazepam (Doral): long acting with a half-life of 39 to 73 hours

Benzodiazepine receptor agonists: Non-Benzodiazepines

- Zaleplon (Sonata): very short acting with a half-life of 1 hour
- Zolpidem Titrate (Ambien): short acting with a half-life of approximately 2.5 to 2.9 hours
- Zolpidem Titrate-CR (Ambien-CR): extended release tables with a half-life of about 2.8 hours
- Eszopiclone (Lunesta): intermediate acting with a half-life of 6 to 9 hours

Melatonin receptor agonist

- Ramelteon (Rozerem): short acting with a half-life of 1 to 3 hours follow these recommendations, there may be serious adverse effects such as sleepwalking, confusional arousals and falls because partial arousals trigger these events. These side effects may occur after taking any sleeping medications and, therefore, the rules must be strictly followed. Also, you should not use a dose higher than the recommended amount prescribed by your physician.

Non-pharmacologic or non-drug treatment includes sleep hygiene measures (see Question 56), relaxation therapy and biofeedback, stimulus control therapy, sleep restriction, and patient education about sleep habits, attitudes toward sleep, and cognitive-behavioral therapy (see **Table 6**). Relaxation therapy incorporates progressive muscle relaxation and biofeedback to reduce the arousing stimuli. Stimulus control therapy is directed at discouraging the learned association between the bedroom and wakefulness and reestablishing the bedroom as the major stimulus for sleep. As part of this therapy, patients are advised to follow certain recommendations (see **Table 7**).

Cognitive-Behavioral Therapy addresses dysfunctional beliefs and attitudes about sleep. Cognitive-Behavioral Therapy educates the patient about the realistic views regarding the nature of sleep and alleviates any misconceptions the patient may have about

Cognitive behavioral therapy

Method of addressing dysfunctional beliefs and attitudes about sleep combined with other non-pharmacologic measures.

Table 6   Non-Pharmacologic or Non-Drug Treatment for the Treatment of Insomnia

- Sleep hygiene measures
- Relaxation therapy including biofeedback
- Stimulus control therapy
- Sleep restriction therapy
- Cognitive-behavioral therapy

Table 7   Stimulus Control Treatment

- Go to bed when you are sleepy.
- Do not watch television, eat, or worry while in bed.
- Use the bed only for sleep and intimacy.
- If you are unable to fall asleep within 20 minutes, get out of bed, go into another room, do something relaxing (such as listening to music or reading light books), and then go back to bed when sleepy. These steps can be repeated.
- Wake up at a fixed time each morning including weekends.
- Do not take naps.

sleep. For example, many individuals are under the impression that if they do not have 8 hours of sleep, they cannot function the next day and that will be a disaster for them. This is not true. Each individual's requirement for sleep is different and 7 ½ to 8 hours is just an average figure; many people can get by with 6 hours or less and some may require more than 8 hours of sleep. The important point to emphasize is how the individual functions the next day. If one can function adequately with sufficient energy, vigor and motivation, even if the patient did not have 8 hours of sleep, that is okay and should not be cause for concern. Similarly, if the patient woke up in the middle of the night but then went back to sleep again, that is okay too as long there is no impairment of the next day's function. As stated in Question 1, it is interesting to note that before the advent of light and electricity, sleep pattern in the early days of civilization was not a consolidated monophasic pattern but was broken into two separate periods of about 4 hours in the evening. There was then a period of wakefulness to contemplate, to meditate, to do some chores and then, after a couple of hours, have the second period of sleep. This pattern has of course changed since the discovery of light and electricity but it is okay to wake up for a short period in the middle of the night as long as you can go back

Treatment

to sleep reasonably quickly and function adequately the next day.

54. Should I take over-the-counter sleeping pills for my sleeplessness?

Before seeking to self-medicate, you should find out what is causing your sleeplessness (see Question 19). In most cases, sleeplessness or insomnia is not a disease, but rather a symptom. In a few patients, no definite cause can be found (**idiopathic insomnia**).

Idiopathic

Not associated with other disease and no causes found.

Before taking any over-the-counter (OTC) medications advertised as sleeping pills, you should seek professional help. Most OTC sleeping pills contain antihistamine, which is used in cold and allergy medications. Scientific studies have never definitively proved that these agents act as hypnotics (drugs that promote good sleep). OTC sleeping pills tend to cause mild drowsiness because of the antihistamine. Unfortunately, the effects spill over into the next day, leading to drowsiness, dizziness, and impairment of daytime function. These drugs also have other undesirable side effects, such as dryness of the mouth.

Glaucoma

Eye condition causing increased pressure within the eye, which may lead to blindness if left untreated.

OTC drugs should be used with extreme caution in patients with **glaucoma** (an eye condition causing increased pressure within the eye, which may lead to blindness if left untreated). They should also be used with caution in patients who have urinary symptoms due to enlargement of the prostate gland, which is common in elderly men. OTC sleeping medications should not be consumed with alcohol as this dangerous combination may severely depress the central nervous system, leading to coma or deep unconsciousness. In patients who suffer from chronic lung disease or sleep apnea (see Question 39), the pills may exacerbate their condition. The adverse effects of OTC sleeping medications will be especially intense in the elderly because of impairment of metabolism of the drugs in old age. Despite their common usage, at a recent consensus conference, the National Institute of Health (NIH) expressed serious reservations about the use of OTC sleeping medications and sedative antidepressant preparations and did not recommend their use for insomnia.

55. Should I take melatonin for my sleep problem?

Melatonin is a natural hormone secreted by the **pineal gland**, a small gland that is located deep in the center of the brain. Melatonin secretion is activated by darkness; for this reason, it is sometimes called the "hormone of darkness." Secretion begins to rise in the evening, with maximum secretion occurring between 3:00 and 5:00 A.M. Light suppresses melatonin secretion.

Pineal gland

Gland in the center of the brain which secretes melatonin.

In the United States, synthetic melatonin formulation in a much greater strength than that secreted physiologically by the pineal gland is available as a nutritional supplement. Its sale is not controlled by the Food and Drug Administration (FDA), which regulates all prescription drugs in the USA. The synthetic melatonin comes in various strengths, but one cannot be certain about the actual amount of melatonin content in each capsule (or whether a particular capsule actually contains any melatonin). This drug has been advertised not only as a sleeping drug, but also as a "magic bullet" capable of curing a variety of illnesses. The limited scientific studies conducted to date have demonstrated that melatonin may have a mild hypnotic effect. In some studies, it has been shown to be beneficial in jet lag syndrome, sleep problems related to shift work, and some other circadian rhythm sleep disorders. Its effect on jet lag syndrome, however, remains controversial. In a small subgroup of elderly patients with complaints of insomnia, melatonin blood levels were found to be subnormal; insomnia in these individuals improved after nightime administration of melatonin.

Absolutely no scientific evidence exists to prove that melatonin is useful in any other medical conditions— contrary to the claims made in magazines and on the Internet. It should also be remembered that melatonin is a hormone, and we do not know its long-term effects on the body. Further scientific studies are needed before this drug could be recommended as a hypnotic agent. The indiscriminate use of melatonin should be discouraged until we know more about it. Melatonin must not be used by pregnant women or nursing mothers.

56. Are there any common-sense measures that I can follow for my sleep problem?

Common-sense measures consist of a set of rules intended to help you maintain a healthy sleep-wake schedule. These steps, also known as sleep hygiene measures (**Table 8**), are detailed here.

Maintain a regular sleep-wake schedule during both weekdays and weekends. Go to bed at a fixed time and wake up at a fixed time. Use an alarm clock if necessary.

Table 8   Sleep Hygiene Measures

- Keep a regular sleep-wake schedule, including weekends.
- Sleep the amount needed to feel rested.
- Avoid napping during the daytime.
- Do not watch television, listen to loud music or plan the next day's activities while in bed.
- Avoid caffeinated beverages (coffee, tea, cola, hot chocolate) in the evening.
- Avoid alcohol near bedtime (i.e., no "night-cap").
- Avoid smoking, especially in the evening.
- Do not go to bed hungry.
- Adjust the bedroom environment.
- Exercise regularly for at least 20 minutes, but do not exercise close to bedtime.

Treatment

Develop a routine for sleep preparation. Eliminate any activities that are incompatible with sleep. Restrict time in bed and go to bed only when you are sleepy. You should stay in bed only for the actual sleep time plus an extra 15 to 20 minutes that may be needed to fall asleep.

As a rule, you should avoid napping during the daytime. Short naps, however, are good for those suffering from narcolepsy. Conversely, napping is counterproductive for those suffering from insomnia.

Do not watch television, listen to loud music, or plan the next day's activities while in bed. Do not use caffeinated beverages (coffee, tea, colas, hot chocolate) in the evening—these drinks will stimulate the arousal system. Discontinue consumption of caffeine after 4:00 P.M. (the half-life of caffeine is about three hours). Avoid alcohol in the evening (no night cap). Although alcohol may help you fall asleep, declining levels of alcohol will produce withdrawal effects, causing rebound awakening and restless sleep. Alcohol also reduces the dream stage of sleep and may cause rebound of REM sleep later at night, triggering nightmares as the level of alcohol falls.

Do not smoke in the evening; nicotine stimulates the central nervous system. Do not have a heavy dinner, but do not go to bed hungry. A heavy meal interferes with sleep by putting an extra strain on the digestive system. Do not wake up to snack or drink in the middle of the night, and restrict fluid intake in the evening.

Do not exercise close to bedtime. You should, however, participate in a regular exercise program, preferably five to six hours before bedtime. Do not keep the room temperature too hot or too cold. Avoid excessive noise or light in the bedroom. Do not use a too-hard or too-soft mattress.

Herbal medicines have been used around the world throughout the ages. Examples of herbal products used to treat sleeplessness and nervous tension include valerian root, ginkgo biloba, linden (lime flower), skull cap, and passion flower.

57. My friend has been using herbal products for sleeplessness. Should I use alternative medicines such as ginkgo biloba, valerian root, and other herbal products?

Herbal medicines have been used around the world throughout the ages. Examples of herbal products used to treat sleeplessness and nervous tension include valerian root, ginkgo biloba, linden (lime flower), skull cap, and passion flower.

Many herbal products have a mild tranquilizing and sedative effect. Such products (such as valerian root and ginkgo biloba) can be bought at health food stores without any prescription, beause they are considered nutritional supplements. With continuous use, herbal products have similar effects to those of sleeping pills used on a long-term basis. That is, herbal products have mild sedative effects but may also cause daytime sedation; their effects will wear off after long-term use. It is also possible to become addicted to such supplements, although this has not been proven.

The problem with herbal products is that most of them did not undergo rigorous scientific study to determine their effectiveness (and, as stated previously, their effectiveness may wane over time in any event). If a person is also taking traditional medications, the herbal products could potentially interact with these drugs. A major concern is that the long-term consequences of most herbal products remain unknown.

Alternative therapy consists of practices that do not rely on traditional medical treatment. Although it is used as a free-standing therapy, it may sometimes be used to complement traditional medical practice. The idea is to strengthen the mind and body, which are interrelated. A tense, stressful mind will indirectly affect the physical aspects of our bodies, and physical illness in turn will affect our minds and emotions. This idea forms the principle of mind-body interaction. Alternative therapy is thought to help fight disease by strengthening the mind and relieving inner tension; however, rigorous scientific evidence is lacking. It may combine several remedies, including exercise, massage, herbal medicines, acupuncture, aromatherapy, meditation, and relaxation techniques. Massage, relaxation exercise, and meditation are, of course, very relaxing to the body and mind and often helpful in patients with chronic insomnia. Most people gain some benefit—at least initially—from alternative therapy, though the effects may not always last long.

Alternative therapy consists of practices that do not rely on traditional medical treatment.

Before beginning any alternative therapy, you should see a sleep specialist, who will first try to find a cause for your sleep problem and suggest appropriate treatment. It is not advisable to use alternative treatment without first thoroughly understanding the source of your sleep problem, because the consequences may be serious. For example, if your excessive sleepiness results from sleep apnea, using alternative therapy instead of the traditional treatment may have disastrous consequences (see Question 39). Similarly, insomnia may be caused by some underlying physical condition; therefore, finding the cause and treating it is the first step in recovery. Alternative therapy may prove useful in some cases of insomnia where no cause is found and the individual is reluctant to use traditional sleep medications for a long time.

58. Why can't I use sleeping medications for sleeplessness for a long time?

Several scientific studies have shown that chronic use of sleeping medications does not help with sleeplessness. On the contrary, in questionnaire-based studies that followed more than 1 million participants for six years such use was associated with increasing harmful effects. In addition, the chances of death in chronic users of prescribed sleeping medications were found to be about three times higher than the risks faced by people not using such sleeping medications. Clearly, this finding is controversial. What is needed to settle the issue is a prospective study comparing a **placebo** (an inactive substance used in a control experiment to reinforce a patient's expectation of obtaining relief) with prescription sleeping medications.

Placebo

Inactive substance used in control experiment to reinforce a patient's expectation of obtaining result.

Sleeping medications are hypnotics that can impair reaction time, daytime performance, judgment, and work efficiency, after either short- or long-term use. Such hypnotic use is associated with more adverse effects in elderly subjects than in younger individuals. In particular, older people are more likely to become injured through falls and to get involved in automobile accidents after using sleeping medications for a long time. Recent investigators have suggested that it is the insomnia rather than the sleeping medications which is responsible for the falls of elderly people. This question of a relationship between insomnia, sleeping medications and falls in the elderly has not been satisfactorily resolved and most likely both of these factors are responsible for the falls.

After long-term use, sleeping medications may lose their effectiveness. There is a general tendency to increase the dose under these circumstances, but the effectiveness of the agent still wanes over time. A sudden withdrawal of such medication after chronic use may cause rebound insomnia which means worsening of sleep dysfunction when the medication is stopped abruptly. This should be differentiated from the more serious withdrawal syndrome observed following sudden withdrawal of medication after long-term use and is characterized by anxiety, tremulousness, more marked insomnia, and severe impairment of performance. There are reports of physical dependence during long-term use of sleeping medications. Adequate studies, however, have not been performed to know the exact frequency of dependence and addiction. **Tolerance**, defined as a reduction in the effect of a drug when administered for a long time and a need for higher doses to produce adequate effect, has often been cited as a potential concern, but this has not been a problem

Sleeping medications are hypnotics that can impair reaction time, daytime performance, judgment, and work efficiency, after either short- or long-term use.

Treatment

Tolerance
Reduction in effect of a drug and need for higher doses to produce adequate effect.

in most of the studies spanning over several weeks in duration. However, its occurrence after long-term use has not been adequately studied.

Anecdotal reports of benefits from long-term use of sleeping medications have been noted, though many of these results may reflect placebo effects. Without scientific study using both the drug and a placebo in a blinded manner, no credence can be given to such reports. In summary, long-term use of sleeping medication is not advisable for two reasons: because of the lack of clear evidence supporting the claims of beneficial effect on sleep architecture and sleep duration; and because of the tendency of the drugs to produce adverse effects, including withdrawal effects, addiction, and increasing probability of mortality. In a small sub-group of insomnia patients who have suffered from insomnia since childhood and without any comorbid condition or any clear evidence of association with another disease, hypnotic medication, particularly the benzodiazepine receptor agonist may have to be used as a long-term treatment.

59. My sleep specialist diagnosed sleep apnea for my daytime sleepiness and snoring, and suggested that I use a nasal mask, which will deliver air from the outside to keep my upper airway passage open. What is this device supposed to do?

Continuous positive airway pressure (CPAP)

Remedial therapy involving a small portable machine used to deliver air through the nose to the back of the throat.

A nasal mask delivers **continuous positive airway pressure (CPAP)** through the nose. It consists of a small, portable machine, which can sit on a lamp table by the side of the bed. The **CPAP device** comprises the following components: a face mask, head straps, a tube or hose connecting a pressure generator or a blower, and a valve to adjust the pressure of the air delivered through the nose into the back of the throat.

With this device, the air from outside, which is delivered at a positive pressure, separates the back of the throat from the uvula, soft palate, and tongue. The column of air acts as a pneumatic splint to keep the airway passage open during sleep. As a consequence, despite excessive reduction of muscle tone in the throat and tongue, outside air continues to flow into the lungs. The patient breathes normally, oxygen levels in the blood do not fall, and snoring is eliminated because no turbulence results from narrowing of the air passage. The patient sleeps soundly, without any apnea-related repeated interruptions. He or she does not feel excessively sleepy in the daytime and, as a result, feels energetic and active and does not complain of fatigue, lack of concentration, forgetfulness, or impotence in men.

Patients must wear the nasal mask device every night during sleep; otherwise, the symptoms will recur. Hence, CPAP treatment is not a cure but rather gives symptomatic relief. The device may be uncomfortable in the beginning, but approximately 75 percent of patients become used to it in the course of two to three weeks. Some individuals may complain of difficulty breathing when the same pressure is delivered during both inhalation and **expiration** (exhaling the air). For such patients, the CPAP device can be adjusted so that it delivers high-pressure air during inspiration and lower-pressure air during expiration, causing bi-level delivery of positive airway pressure (BiPAP).

CPAP device

A small portable machine consisting of a generator and a valve adjusting the pressure of the air delivered through a hose and a face mask into the back of the throat.

Treatment

Expiration

Exhaling air during breathing.

Dorothy comments:

It is hard to believe that I have been wearing a mask connected to a BiPAP (see above) since September 2006 for my sleep apnea (see Question 39). Every night I wear my mask to bed and it has been beneficial in my everyday life. I am now 68 years old and about 7 to 8 months ago, I started having difficulty staying awake during the daytime. I remember on several occasions when I was driving to the bank or Dunkin' Donuts, I would feel very sleepy unless I got out of the car immediately. On many occasions, I would doze off sitting in the car in the parking lot listening to the radio or watching people walk by. On 3 or 4 occasions, passersby knocked on my window and asked me if I was okay and every time I told them I was okay and quickly got out of the car to complete my errands. I talked to my psychologist who was concerned and referred me to a medical doctor who in turn suggested that I go to a sleep center for an evaluation. At the sleep center, the specialist asked me pertinent questions and examined me, and he ordered an overnight sleep study (see Question 37). I went to the sleep laboratory in the evening and the technologist greeted me and explained the procedure to me. The technologist then put wires on my head and various parts of the body to monitor brain waves, breathing patterns, snoring, blood oxygen levels and muscle activities. The technologist was watching my sleep and breathing patterns throughout the night on the monitor. I had another appointment with the sleep specialist to discuss the results of my sleep test. I was told I was not getting an adequate and restful sleep because of my breathing problems during sleep. The doctor made the diagnosis of sleep apnea which was mild but I also have high blood pressure and diabetes mellitus which are risk factors for sleep apnea and the doctor suggested CPAP or BiPAP for me. Therefore, I made another appointment for an overnight sleep study so that a decision can be made about the pressure and the type of mask I need. The technician started me on a CPAP machine with a mask but during the night she changed it to a BiPAP (see above). Because I was having some difficulty exhaling and, therefore, my pressure breathing in was higher and the pressure breathing out was lower and that was comfortable for me. The next day, the doctor sent a prescription with the appropriate pressure to an outside vendor. Someone from the company came and explained to me how the machine worked and how to use it and take care of it daily. It took me a few days to get used to wearing a mask on my face but I have no problems wearing it now, especially knowing how helpful this has been to me. I have also been trying to lose weight because it will help my sleep and breathing as well as my general health. I have been trying to watch my diet and have been visiting the YMCA in our community center 5 days a week. As a result, I have lost a few pounds already. I sleep all night every night wearing my mask. I believe now I am experiencing sleep the way I am supposed to be and I am having deeper and more restful sleep. I no longer fall asleep in the parking lots. I definitely believe wearing the mask has improved my sleep and the quality of my life, thanks to the sleep specialist and all the technical and other professional staff at the sleep center.

60. What are some problems associated with the use of a CPAP machine and a mask delivering air from outside continuously to keep my airway passage open?

The patient may encounter several problems with CPAP, but most can be corrected. Some patients become very uncomfortable—even claustrophobic—when using the nasal mask. In most cases, explanation

The patient may encounter several problems with CPAP, but most can be corrected.

and assurance suffice to relieve their anxiety. If the mask is not tightly fitted, the air may leak around the edges, irritating the skin of the face and the eyes. Some people complain of dryness and stuffiness of the nose, which can be improved by attaching a humidifier (delivering warm or cold moist air; however, warm air would be preferable) to the CPAP machine. If the mask is too tight, it may cause chafing of the bridge of the nose. The solution is to loosen the head gear slightly and use a soft pad over the bridge of the nose. If these measures fail, then a different type of mask may be used with benefit. Recently, there has been considerable improvement in mask design by different companies and a variety of masks which are suitable for different people are now available and, therefore, there is a choice now. If one mask is not agreeable with a particular patient, then that patient can choose from several other types of masks and nasal pillows.

Some people complain of dryness of the mouth because of mouth breathing; in these cases, the best choice is to use a full face mask covering the nose and the mouth. Several types of full face masks are available. Some patients, however, may become claustrophobic with these devices and in these people, a chin strap to keep the mouth shut, along with a nasal mask may help. Some patients—particularly those suffering from nasal allergy—may complain of nasal congestion and a runny nose. In these patients, nasal decongestant drops may prove helpful.

Other problems may include psychological worries about the patient's relationship with his or her bed partner and a feeling of invalidity. The bed partner may also be psychologically disturbed by the prospect of sleeping with a person who is wearing a mask and head gear, resembling a man or woman from outer space. A thoughtful discussion with both bed partners will allay such psychological fears. It is very important to explain to the patient before treating with a **CPAP titration** about the various problems and how to correct them and the advantages of CPAP. A follow-up by telephone after a week of CPAP titration in the laboratory is important to find out how the patient is doing. Also, a follow-up visit about one month and three months after the CPAP titration is important so that the physician and the patient can discuss any problems and how to go about solving the problems. Adequate and early communication between the patient and the sleep specialist is the key to compliance with CPAP.

CPAP titration

Gradually adjusting the flow of air until the desired effect is achieved.

Treatment

61. Do I have options other than a mask treatment (CPAP) for my sleep apnea problem?

Unfortunately, there are no effective medications available to treat the problems in the upper airway and, therefore, to treat sleep apnea. In patients with mild to moderate sleep apnea as judged by the sleep specialist based on the history, physical findings and overnight sleep study, some other options may be tried but the numerous studies, including the follow-up studies, have shown benefit in about 50% of the patients. Many of these patients again developed snoring and all the other symptoms of sleep apnea after initial improvement following these other options. Patients with a risk factor such as associated high blood pressure, or with a history of heart attack or stroke, should ideally be treated with CPAP titration rather than the other options because there is a good chance of improvement and correction of abnormal breathing events following CPAP, thus minimizing the chances of recurrence of heart attack or stroke in most of these cases.

Other options, such as oral appliances and upper airway surgery, may be selected for patients who cannot tolerate CPAP treatment or for those with mild to moderate sleep apnea as defined above without any associated risk factors. The oral appliances include jaw advancement devices which increase the airway space in the back of the throat, thus promoting smooth airflow in and out of the lungs during sleep. Another appliance is a lower jaw (mandible) repositioning splint; however, we do not know the long-term benefits and side effects of these devices. Furthermore, some patients complain of excessive salivation (drooling), dryness of the mouth, **temporomandibular joint** pain, discomfort of the teeth and facial muscle pain. Another device which has been tried in some patients is called a tongue retaining device to pull the tongue forward and hold it in a position which will open the airway space in the back of the throat, but this is not effective in most patients and many patients find it uncomfortable and painful.

Temporomandibular joint

The jaw joint.

Some upper airway surgical procedures are available such as surgery on the soft palate (tongue like projection from the roof of the mouth in the back of the throat) and other tissues surrounding this soft palate. This can be performed either by actual surgical resection using a scalpel or by laser technique, or the reduction of the volume of the soft palate and other tissues surrounding it can be achieved using radio frequency technique. These surgeries will cause severe pain in the immediate post-operative period and there may be some alteration of the voice and some regurgitation of fluids through the nose. Another surgery on the palate is called palatal implant or **Pillar procedure** in which rods made of polyester material are implanted into the soft palate to prevent the collapse of the palate and narrowing of the upper airway in the back of the throat when the muscle tone falls during sleep. This procedure is helpful in some patients; but in other patients the problem is not in the region of the palate but in the lower part of the airway, in which case this procedure would not be helpful. Several patients have undergone nasal surgery to remove nasal polyps or to correct nasal septum defects. Evidence of benefit from this surgery is lacking.

All patients who suffer from sleep apnea should of course follow some lifestyle changes such as loss of weight in overweight patients by controlling the diet and by regular exercise. However, in massively obese patients, these measures may not be helpful and they may have to undergo some special procedures, such as **bariatric surgery,** which may be helpful in achieving weight loss but which have long-term side effects. The patient should also stop smoking because there is a clear relationship between smoking and prevalence of sleep apnea syndrome. However, whether stopping smoking will improve the sleep apnea remains to be determined. The patient should definitely avoid alcohol in the evening and avoid sleeping pills which will worsen sleep apnea.

Pillar procedure

Surgery on the palate in which polyester rods are implanted into the soft palate.

Bariatric surgery

Procedure performed to assist obese patients in achieving weight loss.

Treatment

62. How is narcolepsy treated?

The treatment of narcolepsy includes both drug and non-drug therapies. The physician may prescribe central nervous system stimulants for sleep attacks and sleepiness, carefully monitoring the dose, the progress

The treatment of narcolepsy includes both drug and non-drug therapies.

of the illness, and any side effects of the medication. The most commonly used drugs are Ritalin, amphetamines, and a new drug called Modafinil (Provigil). Because of their potential for abuse, use of such medications must be closely monitored by the physician. Modafinil (Provigil), because of its better side effect profile, is usually the first line of stimulant drug used for excessive sleepiness in narcolepsy. Listen to what Filomena has to say:

Having been properly diagnosed and under medical care, my life has been given back. I am no longer afraid to drive myself or others on long trips. I recently drove from Virginia to Pennsylvania without any worries of falling asleep. I feel alert and reborn. I have gained control of a part of me that I had no control of for many years. The Provigil, when taken properly, allows me to function. I have learned how to take the medication properly for my lifestyle. I can now watch my favorite TV shows from beginning to end. So far, I have not experienced any side effects from the medication and have only reaped the benefits. I am able to go to sleep at night with very little resistance—the one and only perk of having narcolepsy. My mother once told me, 'You control your body, don't let your body control you.' I can honestly say I can now control my body.

Drug therapies for cataplexy, sleep paralysis, and vivid hallucinatory dreams include antidepressant agents. Another drug which has become available recently is Gamma Hydroxybutyrate (Xyrem) which is used to control symptoms of cataplexy, hallucinations and sleep paralysis for patients who do not respond to the antidepressant agents including the newer selective serotonin reuptake inhibitors (SSRIs).

Non-drug treatments for narcolepsy involve following general sleep hygiene measures, which are common-sense measures (see Question 56) intended to regularize the sleep schedule, supplemented by short daytime naps. Scheduling short sleep periods (lasting 20 to 30 minutes) during the daytime may help temporarily prevent sleep attacks and sleepiness. Joining a narcolepsy support group may aid the patient in understanding the disease and coping with his or her problem. Untreated patients with narcolepsy must avoid driving and occupations dealing with heavy equipment. It is important for patients to address lifestyle and behavior. These patients should have counseling for the purpose of educating family members as well as school teachers about the disorder. Some adjustments and accommodations in the classroom and employment may be needed.

63. I wake up with terrible leg cramps in the middle of the night. What should I do?

Most people describe leg cramps as painful, crampy sensations in the legs, usually affecting the calf muscles and occuring in the middle of the night. Colloquially, these events are described as "Charlie horses". They often cause problems with sleep maintenance and may occasionally be associated with daytime sleepiness. Episodes are more common in older individuals than in younger ones. Leg cramps are usually unilateral, affecting one leg at a time.

An occasional leg cramp at night, waking a person from sleep once in a while, may not cause much sleep disturbance and may not be associated with any significant underlying disorder. Before trying any measures to relieve the leg cramps, however, it is important to determine whether an underlying cause is present. Frequent leg cramps, occurring not only during the night but also during the daytime, may suggest that another disorder is at work. Therefore, the affected individual should consult a professional, who will try to identify the cause of this complaint. Once a cause is found, treatment should be directed at the underlying problem, which will generally relieve the leg cramps.

Sources of leg cramps may include a variety of general medical disorders (e.g., kidney failure, low blood sodium and calcium, heart failure, arthritis, reduced function of the thyroid and parathyroid glands, diabetes mellitus), neurological disorders (e.g., Lou Gehrig's disease, diseases of the nerves innervating the muscles in the legs, Parkinson's disease, muscle diseases), and drug-induced cramps (e.g., after ingestion of lipid-lowering agents or diuretics that help produce urine). Many pregnant women also complain of cramps in the later stages of pregnancy. In addition, vigorous exercise is associated with cramps. Finally, a rare form of familial cramping exists.

When all these causes are excluded, there remains a group of individuals complaining of nighttime leg cramps of unknown origin. Treatment for these patients consists of both drug and non-drug therapy. Stretching and massaging the legs and bending the foot upward may help. If these non-drug treatments fail, a small dose of quinine sulfate may be administered to patients who experience disabling nocturnal cramps. Consult with a physician before using quinine, because this drug may have undesirable side effects. In any case, pregnant women and patients with liver disease must avoid quinine.

PART FIVE

Living with a Sleep Disorder

64. What happens if I am sleep deprived?

Sleep deprivation (partial or complete) experiments have been conducted in both humans and animals. In rats, complete sleep deprivation lasting for 10 to 30 days caused the animals to lose temperature control and weight despite increase in food intake; eventually, the rats died. In 1965, a 17-year-old California student named Randy Gardner tried to set a world record by staying awake for 264 hours and 12 minutes. He then slept for 14 hours and 40 minutes without any permanent adverse effects. During the sleep deprivation experiment, Gardner was, however, drifting into transient periods of NREM stage 1 (see Question 1) known as **microsleep.**

Sleep deprivation causes fatigue; sleepiness; deterioration of performance, attention, and motivation; and diminishment of mental concentration and intellectual capacity.

Sleep deprivation causes fatigue; sleepiness; deterioration of performance, attention, and motivation; and diminishment of mental concentration and intellectual capacity. It also increases the chances of accidents at work and during driving. Thus, sleep deprivation lowers the quality of life and jeopardizes both personal and public safety. Sleep deprivation may have been responsible for many national and international catastrophes (as described in the Introduction). There is clear recent evidence that sleep deprivation may increase morbidity (chances of becoming ill) and obesity by changing the body's metabolism. Sleep deprivation may also cause an impairment of intellect, memory and judgment (see Question 65).

65. Can sleeplessness cause adverse physical and mental effects?

Every individual has a certain minimum requirement for sleep (see Question 3). If this minimum sleep requirement is not met, symptoms of insomnia will interfere with the person's life and efficiency at work. These symptoms may include irritability, lack of concentration, tiredness, sleepiness in the daytime, and temporary forgetfulness. All the symptoms related to insomnia may interfere with creativity and judgment. There are also indications that sleeplessness may interfere with long-term memory and intellect. An early epidemiologic study showed an increasing chance of death from coronary arterial disease, cancer or stroke in those who sleep less than 4 hours per night and this study has been confirmed by recent observations. However, other factors, such as sleeping medications, may have been responsible for some of the adverse effects thought to be related to insomnia. There is, therefore, no clear cut conclusion yet. However, sleep deprivation experiments, in both humans and animals, have clearly shown adverse physical and mental effects related to sleep deprivation. In addition to the short-term effects of sleep disturbance on inadequate functioning during the daytime, patients who suffer from chronic insomnia have shown impaired work performance and productivity, reduced social and physical functioning and reduced overall quality of life. There is also an increased risk for developing subsequent depression associated with significant suicidal behavior (see Question 82). There are suggestions of increased morbidity and mortality from increasing automobile accidents, coronary arterial disease, high blood pressure, obesity and diabetes mellitus.

66. Can a person either become sick or die after complete sleep deprivation?

It is impossible, from both ethical and practical stand-points, to completely sleep-deprive a human. During sleep deprivation experiments in humans, researchers have noted the occurrence of frequent periods of "microsleep." Subjects have been found to doze repeatedly with transient periods of stage 1 NREM sleep (see Question 1), with heaviness or drooping of the eyelids and sagging of the head.

In an earlier experiment, subjects who awakened after REM sleep deprivation were thought to experience hallucinations and other psychotic features; these findings could not be replicated in later experiments, however. An increased amount of slow wave and dream (REM) sleep does take place in the recovery period after sleep deprivation.

Animals subjected to total sleep deprivation will die. This finding was observed by Rechtschaffen and colleagues in their sleep deprivation experiments with rats (see Question 64).

Sleep deprivation experiments in humans, as well as epidemiological studies, have clearly shown serious adverse effects on the physical and mental health of an individual. Sleep deprivation, either as a result of lifestyle changes or primary sleep disorders, increases the mortality and morbidity (increased chances of sickness). Sleep deprivation causes a **decrement** of the appetite suppressant (leptin) but an **increment** of the appetite-stimulating (ghrelin) hormone causing increased body weight and obesity. Sleep deprivation is

Decrement

To subtract or reduce, as observed in certain chemicals during sleep deprivation.

Increment

To increase or add, as observed in certain chemicals during sleep deprivation.

also associated with diabetes mellitus, increased prevalence of heart disease due to coronary arterial disease. One of the causative factors for increased prevalence of obesity in the USA may be sleep deprivation. The National Sleep Foundation poll of 2002 polling America showed that 39% of adults slept less than 7 hours a night. Several studies have also shown increased lapses of attention and vigilance and impairment of memory and executive functioning which may be responsible for increased frequency of accidents and motor vehicle crashes and accidental deaths. Sleep deprivation is also thought to be associated with depression. In some studies, both long and short durations of sleep have been associated with increased morbidity and mortality.

67. Is it harmful if someone sleeps more than his or her usual requirement of sleep? In other words, does an excessive amount of sleep cause any adverse effects on the human mind and body?

To answer this question, you must know your normal requirement for sleep. This optimal amount of sleep will make you feel refreshed the next day so that you can function in an efficient manner. If you sleep for a shorter period than your normal requirement, you will suffer adverse consequences as a result of sleep deprivation (see Question 64). If you have a primary sleep disorder, such as narcolepsy (see Question 42) or sleep apnea (see Question 39), you will sleep excessively during the daytime. Short naps may be beneficial in narcolepsy, but do not help patients with sleep apnea.

There have been reports in the past which indicated that an extended amount of sleep can have adverse effects. In other words, if a person sleeps for an excessive amount of time (that is, in excess of the usual requirement of night sleep), his or her functional capacity the next day may be reduced and work efficiency may be impaired. In such a case, the test for vigilance may also be impaired and reaction time prolonged the next day. In addition, the individual may suffer from poor cognition and depressed mood following an extended period of sleep. Sometimes, one may suffer from the "Rip Van Winkle effect," which is characterized by exhaustion and irritability the next day after prolonged night sleep. Whether one can extend the amount of sleep in absence of a sleep debt remains, however, controversial. Most modern sleep investigators believe that extra sleep simply means repaying sleep debt. It is not really possible to obtain extra sleep once the subject's usual daily sleep requirement is met. Studies do not support an impairment after extra sleep or after too much sleep.

The best advice is to restrict your sleep time to the amount that makes you feel invigorated and efficient the next day. One study found an increased incidence of death from coronary arterial disease, stroke, or cancer in both individuals who sleep more than 10 hours and individuals who sleep less than four hours. The results of this study, however, remain controversial.

68. Is snoring related to any physical defect, and can snoring cause any physical illness or memory impairment?

The answer to Question 74 discusses the causes of snoring. In addition to physical defects in the throat, other defects that may contribute to snoring include a receding chin, a large tongue, and a thick neck. Furthermore, nasal congestion, nasal allergy or nasal septum defects may promote mouth-breathing which will generate increased turbulence in the back of the throat, contributing to the snoring. It has been suggested that loud snoring for a long time may lead to mild swelling of the soft palate and uvula and may cause damage to the nerves supplying these structures as a result of the repeated vibrations associated with snoring. This theory, however, remains controversial. In the early epidemiological studies, snoring has been cited as a risk factor for causing high blood pressure or coronary artery disease, or even stroke, but most of those patients with snoring probably were associated with sleep apnea which may cause serious long-term consequences such as high blood pressure, stroke or coronary artery disease (see Question 70). There have been some suggestions that snoring may disturb the sleep, repeatedly waking the patient and causing fragmentation of sleep. This may lead to excessive daytime sleepiness and possibly some interference with concentration and attention in the daytime. Early memory impairment in patients with snoring may actually be related to an associated sleep apnea which causes blood oxygen level to fall repeatedly during sleep at night rather than to snoring itself. There is another way snoring may cause sleep disturbance. Snoring, of course, will disturb the bed partner who may decide to wake up the snoring person briefly or encourage him to change position from the supine to the side, thus causing sleep disturbances throughout the night, and the interruptions in sleep may cause excessive daytime sleepiness, irritability and lack of concentration.

69. Does sleep disturbance affect organs in the body?

It has traditionally been said that sleep is a function of the brain and that any disturbance of sleep will solely affect the brain. Many studies have proved this point. Sleep disturbance does affect brain function, causing sleeplessness, excessive sleepiness, or abnormal timing of sleep and sometimes affecting attention, concentration, intellect, and memory.

Until very recently, however, researchers had largely neglected the effects of sleep disturbance on organs and systems of the body other than the brain. There is now a keen interest in understanding how sleep problems influence general health and other systems of the body. An important recent study has shown that chronic sleep loss has harmful effects on the metabolism of carbohydrates and hormone regulation—particularly, blood sugar, thyroid function, and cortisone secretion.

Investigations of circadian rhythm disorders in shift workers have clearly shown that the resulting sleep disruption has adverse effects on the digestive system, including development of stomach ulcers. As discussed in Questions 64 and 65, sleep deprivation experiments in humans, as well as epidemiological studies, have clearly shown serious adverse effects on different body systems and organs.

It has traditionally been said that sleep is a function of the brain and that any disturbance of sleep will solely affect the brain.

There is now a keen interest in understanding how sleep problems influence general health and other systems of the body.

70. My friend told me that sleep apnea is a serious condition, which may cause stroke, heart disease, and high blood pressure. Is my friend correct?

Your friend is absolutely correct. There is an increased association between sleep apnea and stroke, heart disease (irregular heart rhythm and narrowing of the coronary arteries that supply blood to the heart), and high blood pressure. The question of whether sleep apnea by itself or obesity, high blood cholesterol, diabetes mellitus, alcoholism and smoking (all of which are risk factors for stroke, heart disease, high blood pressure, and sleep apnea) are actually responsible for an increased association of these diseases remains somewhat controversial. Most investigators believe that sleep apnea is an important risk factor for all of these conditions. Approximately 50% of patients with sleep apnea have high blood pressure, whereas 30% of patients with high blood pressure have sleep apnea. Epidemiological studies have clearly shown the relationship between high blood pressure and degree of sleep apnea (that is, how many times a person stops breathing per hour of sleep).

71. I have heard that people with sleep apnea may die suddenly in the middle of the night. Is this true?

Several reports have suggested that sudden death in sleep apnea patients may occur in the middle and late part of the night, or in the early hours of the morning. This problem has been reported in patients who suffer from severe sleep apnea, which is associated with repeated prolonged apneas, dangerously low blood oxygen levels, irregular heart rhythms, sleep disruption, and excessive daytime sleepiness. For this reason, it is important to see a physician when symptoms suggest sleep apnea in order to prevent long-term complications affecting the heart, brain, and circulatory system that could potentially elevate one's blood pressure and even cause sudden death.

72. Can sleeplessness lead to psychological or psychiatric problems, cause someone to develop a psychopathic personality, or even lead a person to commit murder or practice other violent behaviors?

A close interrelationship exists between chronic insomnia and psychiatric problems. In several surveys and studies, researchers have found that insomnia commonly coexists or precedes the onset of a number of psychiatric illnesses. The psychiatric conditions most commonly associated with insomnia include depression and anxiety. Major psychiatric illness, such as schizophrenia, may cause insomnia or **hypersomnia** as well. Individuals with insomnia are much more likely to develop a new psychiatric disorder, particularly major depression, within 6 to 12 months of the onset of their sleeplessness. It should also be remembered that individuals with insomnia often complain of anxiety and depression.

Most insomniacs do not develop a psychopathic personality. Conversely, a person with a psychopathic personal-

Hypersomnia

Recurrent episodes of excessive daytime sleepiness or prolonged nighttime sleep.

ity may suffer from sleeplessness. Insomnia does not lead to homicidal or violent behaviors unlike some other sleep problems, such as sleepwalking (see Question 73).

73. Can one perform complex acts and behave violently or even commit murder during sleepwalking episodes?

Several reports of sleep-related violence, including homicide, suicide and other types of aggression, have appeared in professional journals, in print media, and on radio and television. Violent behavior during sleep is a symptom of many underlying disorders, but not by itself a disease.

The question of whether one can perform complex acts, behave violently, or even commit murder during sleepwalking episodes (see Question 78) continues to inspire heated debate. Following sleepwalking episodes, subjects usually do not remember the events (except for fragments of memory of the spells) and there is no conscious wakefulness. Therefore, it has been argued that patients who experience these episodes cannot be responsible for their acts. In several court cases involving violence and homicide, in which the defense has claimed sleepwalking and confusional episodes as the culprit, the verdicts have gone both for and against these defendants. In one case in Canada (the "Parks" case), the defendant drove 23 km, killed his mother-in-law, and attempted to kill his father-in-law. The defense argued that the plaintiff was not consciously aware of his behavior during the sleepwalking episode, and he was ultimately acquitted. In another case in Pennsylvania (the "Butler, PA" case), a man who fatally shot his wife used a criminal defense of confusional arousal out of an episode of sleep apnea; he was found guilty.

Besides sleepwalking, two other conditions—**confusional arousals** and sleep terrors—may occur during deep dreamless sleep; complex behaviors without conscious awareness may arise out of these episodes. In addition, violent behavior may occur during the dreaming stage of sleep. It is notable that a high incidence of violent, aggressive behavior occurs in men, implying that testosterone may play a role in such cases.

Certain triggering factors may precipitate violent sleepwalking episodes; it is important to remember them for the purpose of preventing such incidents. These factors include sleep deprivation, exertion, stress, and ingestion of drugs and alcohol.

In addition to arising out of deep dreamless sleep, sleep-related violent behavior and acts may occur secondary to other neurologic, primary sleep disorders and psychiatric disorders. Consequently, the diagnosis should confirm that the violent behavior arises during sleep in the absence of conscious awareness. Guidelines have been developed to identify the role played in violence by a specific sleep disorder. The sleep disorder should be diagnosed through a history or with an overnight **video-polysomnographic study** conducted by a sleep specialist. Each episode must generally last for a few minutes to warrant a diagnosis, and the behavior must be abrupt and without apparent motivation. On regaining consciousness perplexity and a lack of awareness without any attempt to escape are important features. In particular, partial or complete loss of memory for the event is very characteristic of this phenomenon. A sleepwalking episode generally occurs during the first third of the night and may be precipitated by the triggering factors mentioned earlier. It is also important to remember that sleep-related violence is not recurrent.

What is the basis of aggression and rage in this condition? The answer to this question remains unknown. Environmental, social, and genetic factors may all contribute to its **etiology**. The legal implications of the source of such behavior have been discussed and debated by the medical and legal profession without any definite conclusion.

Etiology

Cause of a symptom or condition.

PART SIX

Normal vs. Abnormal Sleep Behavior – which is which?

74. Is snoring a nuisance or a problem?

Before one can answer this question, it is important to know what causes snoring. Snoring is defined as a noisy (mild or loud) resonant breathing during sleep caused by the vibration of the soft tissues in the back of the throat behind the tongue. These soft tissues include the **soft palate** (a soft, muscular tissue in the back of the roof of the mouth), **uvula** (a soft, pear-shaped structure hanging below the soft palate behind the tongue), **tonsils**, back and side walls of the throat, and back of the tongue. **Snoring** is caused mainly by vibration of the uvula and the soft palate.

Snoring can be mild (occasional), moderate (frequent), and severe (very loud and frequent). During sleep, the muscle tone in the back of the throat, including that in the tongue and other muscles in the upper airway passage (through which air goes into the lungs), decreases; and especially marked decrement or absence of muscle tone occurs during the dream stage of sleep (REM sleep). This loss of muscle tone causes the tongue to go toward the back of the throat, slightly narrowing the upper airway and creating turbulence. The turbulence causes vibrations, mainly of the uvula and soft palate, which produce snoring. When a person is lying on his or her back, the tongue tends to go farther back; hence, snoring is worse in this position. In a severe case, snoring occurs in all body positions. Snoring becomes worse when muscle tone is greatly decreased (for example, when we are tired, drink alcohol, or take sleeping medication). In the presence of enlarged tonsils, a large and long uvula, or a bulky soft palate, the upper airway passage is narrowed even further, causing loud snoring. Partial obstruction in the nose (because of a cold or allergy that causes swelling of the tissues,

Soft palate

Soft, muscular tissue in the back of the roof of the mouth.

Uvula

The small piece of soft pear-shaped structure that can be seen dangling down from the soft palate over the back of the tongue.

Tonsils

Areas of lymphoid tissue on either side of the throat.

Snoring

Noisy sound generated by an obstruction to the free flow of air through the passages at the back of the mouth and nose caused by vibration of the uvula and soft palate during sleep, contributing to reduction of sleep quality.

for example, or a nasal septal deviation) may also contribute to snoring.

Snoring affects more men than women, and its prevalence increases with age. An important survey from San Marino, Italy, in the early 1980s found that 60 percent of men older than 60 years and 19 percent of the overall sample were habitual snorers. Later surveys confirmed the high prevalence of snoring in men. Those who smoke, lie on their back, are obese, and are physically inactive were found to be more likely to snore. Individuals with frequent loud snoring (habitual snorers) are more likely to doze off at the wheel and become involved in a traffic accident due to sleepiness and tiredness.

Mild snoring may be a social nuisance. In contrast, loud, frequent, almost nightly snoring may be the forerunner of a more serious disorder with severe long- and short-term consequences. That is, it may be the warning sign of something more sinister. Loud snoring may repeatedly disturb sleep for brief moments throughout the night. Although the snorer will not remember these brief interruptions in sleep, a recording of the electrical activities of the brain (EEG) will indicate recurrent periods of awakenings. Because the snorer does not get an adequate amount of sleep, he or she is sleep-deprived and prone to frequent sleepiness in the daytime. This condition is merely an intermediate stage between snoring and the next stage, when snoring becomes associated with periodic cessation of breathing throughout the night. This stage signifies a more serious condition than simple snoring—the snorer is now suffering from sleep apnea (see Question 39).

Individuals with frequent loud snoring (habitual snorers) are more likely to doze off at the wheel and become involved in a traffic accident due to sleepiness and tiredness.

75. My bed partner snores loudly, driving me crazy. He makes noises like a freight train. He also feels sleepy in the daytime. Should he use a snore guard or see a doctor?

If the snoring is loud enough (like the noise of a freight train) to drive the bed partner crazy, then certainly it is not just a nuisance. Additionally, if the snorer feels extremely sleepy in the daytime, then he or she is experiencing fragmented sleep (repeated brief awakenings at night), which causes daytime sleepiness. This condition may indicate that the individual is developing sleep apnea (see Question 39).

If snoring occurs only when lying on the back, the person should try to sleep on his or her side. If the snoring and daytime sleepiness continue, then the individual should see a doctor for investigation of possible breathing disorders during sleep.

Numerous advertisements tout cures of snoring and sleep-related breathing problems. One should be wary of these anti-snore devices, most of which do not benefit the sufferer or may reduce the intensity of snoring only temporarily. The best advice would be to see a physician, preferably a sleep specialist, who can make a positive diagnosis of breathing disorder during sleep early enough to prevent long-term adverse effects.

76. I am a 20-year-old woman. I wake up in the middle of the night to eat and drink. Is this behavior abnormal?

You may be suffering one of two eating disorders associated with sleep. One is **sleep-related eating disorder**

(SRED) and the other is **nocturnal eating/drinking syndrome.**

SRED is common in women between the ages of 20 and 30. These individuals have recurrent episodes of eating and drinking during partial arousals from deep or slow wave sleep. Generally, these patients do not remember the episodes. Sometimes these patients display strange eating behavior (e.g., consuming inedible or toxic substances such as frozen pizza, raw bacon and cat food). The episodes cause sleep disruption with weight gain and occasionally injury has been reported. These patients often have a history of sleepwalking. The condition can occur without any associated cause or it can be comorbid with other sleep disorders (e.g., sleepwalking, see Question 78, sleep apnea) and hypnotic medications such as benzodiazepines and non-benzodiazepine receptor agonists and other psycho-tropic agents. They should consult a sleep specialist because treatment with medications such as dopaminer-gic agents, antiepileptic drugs or antidepressants will be helpful in many of these patients.

The other condition which should be considered in your case is nocturnal eating syndrome, which is also more common in young women. The individual is fully alert during the episode and can recall the episode the next morning. These individuals wake up repeat-edly during the night to eat and drink, and they have insomnia. More than 50% of their total calories are consumed during the night. Often they experience a craving for carbohydrates, resulting in weight gain. Some may also have an underlying depression. This condition differs from bulimia, which also affects young women. In **bulimia**, the patient has a craving for excessive eating and drinking, characterized by binge eating and often purging and vomiting. Bulimia

Sleep related eating disorder (SRED)

Type of sleep disorder in which people eat while in a state of partial arousal from sound sleep. They may eat in bed or roam through the house and prowl the kitchen.

Nocturnal eating/drinking syndrome

Condition character-ized by awakening in the middle of the night, getting out of bed, and consuming large quantities of food quickly and uncontrollably, then returning to sleep.

Bulimia

Eating disorder char-acterized by cravings for excessive eating and drinking, fol-lowed by purging and vomiting.

127

is not restricted to the night, which differentiates it from nocturnal eating/drinking syndrome. The treatment of nocturnal eating/drinking syndrome consists of behavioral modification, calorie restriction, and sometimes medications.

77. My daughter, aged 15, grinds her teeth at night. Is that normal?

Tooth grinding or tooth crunching (also known as bruxism) commonly occurs in children and young adults between the ages of 10 and 20. In the vast majority of cases, the individual is normal in all other respects. Sometimes tooth grinding is associated with **malocclusion** of the teeth (the upper and lower teeth do not fit well) or with disease of the temporomandibular joint (located in front of the earlobe). The evidence for these associations, however, is not very strong. Children with mental retardation or cerebral palsy frequently develop tooth grinding.

Bruxism involves a vigorous contraction of the muscles of the upper jaw, which rubs the upper and lower teeth against each other. Although it may occur at any stage of sleep, it most commonly takes place in the lighter stages of non-dream sleep and the dream stage of sleep. Tooth grinding produces a characteristic noise that may disturb the bed partner. Repeated episodes of tooth grinding may cause excessive tooth wear and dental decay. Sometimes the patient will complain of facial pain, headache, and pain in the region of the upper jaw. Episodes of tooth grinding are often triggered by stress, anxiety, alcohol consumption, and tooth-related diseases. Occasionally, tooth grinding runs in the family.

Malocclusion

Condition in which the upper and lower teeth do not fit well.

Bruxism

Vigorous contraction of muscles of the upper jaw, which rubs the upper and lower teeth against each other.

Tooth grinding does not require any specific treatment, other than evaluation by a dentist. In severe cases of frequent tooth grinding with evidence of wearing of the teeth, it is advisable to wear a tooth guard to protect the teeth from further damage. If the patient has a high stress or anxiety level, psychotherapy and other counseling may be needed.

78. My son, aged 10 years, wakes up approximately 45 to 60 minutes after going to sleep. He looks confused and then attempts to get out of bed, sometimes walking toward the door and going to the living room. Is sleepwalking normal for his age?

Sleepwalking is normal at this age. Sleepwalking (also known as **somnambulism**) is very common in children, most frequently occurring at an age between 5 and 12 years. Sometimes, it persists into adult life. It rarely begins in adults, however. Most children outgrow sleepwalking, with disappearance of this condition during adolescence.

A sleepwalking episode most commonly occurs during the first third of the night, arising out of the deep, dreamless stage of sleep. The condition is classified as a **partial arousal disorder**, during which the body is apparently active but the brain is confused and only partially awakened. The subject sits up in bed, looks around vacantly, may lie down again or get out of bed, and attempts to walk toward the door. Sometimes he or she may leave the room, climb or descend stairs, and occasionally even go out the front door into the streets.

Somnambulism

Sleepwalking. Very common in children, sometimes persisting into adulthood

Partial arousal disorder

Condition in which the body is apparently active, but the brain is confused and only partially awakened.

129

On most occasions, individuals find their way around the bed and come back to bed to lie down. The subject is not aware of what is going on around him or her, but sometimes may respond to a question, albeit inappropriately. Any attempt to arouse the person fully may make the episode worse, so it is best to help the individual find his or her way around the bed to avoid injury from objects in the room.

Generally, sleepwalking does not cause injury. Occasionally, however, the patient may trip and fall, sustaining an injury. Rarely during the episode of sleepwalking, the subject may engage in violent behavior (see Question 73). Indeed, there have been cases of apparent homicidal incidents during somnambulistic episodes. Any such abnormal behavior during sleepwalking is usually abrupt and without any apparent motivation or premeditation. The individual does not attempt to escape or cover up the action and generally has the appearance of perplexity or horror. He or she will not remember the sleepwalking episodes next morning.

Most commonly, sleepwalking occurs as a single episode lasting as long as 10 minutes (sometimes longer), and occasionally there may be multiple episodes during sleep at night. Episodes are triggered by sleep deprivation, fatigue, concurrent illness (such as fever or diseases for which sedative medications are ingested), and psychological stress. In adults with sleepwalking, there is frequently a history of somnambulism. Sleepwalking episodes run in the family and are often associated with sleep terror (see Question 47). Occurrence of this condition for the first time in adults should lead to a suspicion of an underlying disease, such as sleep apnea or a neurodegenerative disease like Alzheimer's disease.

In most cases, sleepwalking does not require any specific treatment other than reassurance and preventive measures. The bedroom furniture should be readjusted and any bedroom doors should be locked so that the subject cannot leave the room. Also, any hard objects lying in the bedroom should be removed to prevent injury. In severe cases involving frequent episodes of sleepwalking, especially if they are associated with injuries, if the affected individual must spend time with a friend in an unfamiliar environment, then he or she can be temporarily treated with medications, such as a benzodiazepine or a tricyclic antidepressant.

79. I am concerned about my son, aged 1, who has head banging and rocking movements of his body during sleep. Is this an abnormal sleep disorder?

Head banging and rocking movements of the body during sleep, also called **rhythmic movement disorders**, most commonly occur in infants younger than 18 months of age and are occasionally associated with mental retardation. A rhythmic movement disorder can occur at any stage of sleep. It is rarely familial. This condition becomes evident during the transition between sleep and wakefulness and includes three characteristic movements: head banging with forward and backward rhythmic head moments; head rolling wih side-to-side head movemens; and rocking movements of the body.

Rhythmic movement disorder

Benign condition, usually in infants younger than 18 months, and spontaneously outgrown. Sometimes confused with seizures occurring at night.

Rhythmic movement disorder is a benign condition, and the patient will usually outgrow the episodes. Sometimes, the episodes may be confused with seizures occurring at night. If there is any doubt about the diagnosis, professional help should be sought.

80. I am a 22-year-old man. On some nights, especially if I had a stressful day, I get sudden jerking movements of the legs with a sensation of falling as I am about to go to sleep. I am concerned about these symptoms. Am I having a nocturnal seizure or developing a serious neurological illness?

Hypnic jerks

Sudden jerking motions of the legs or whole body occurring at the moment of falling asleep.

Hypnic jerks may occur following a period of stress, fatigue, or sleep deprivation. The only treatment required is an explanation with reassurance.

The condition described here appears to involve **hypnic jerks,** which are normal physiological phenomena affecting as many as 70 percent of all members of the general population. These sudden jerking movements of the legs or the whole body last for a few seconds and always occur at the moment of falling asleep. They are not accompanied by any loss of control of the urinary bladder or tongue biting. The jerking movements generally do not interfere with sleep, although sometimes repeated intense jerking movements may cause anxiety, creating difficulty in getting to sleep. Similar movements may sometimes occur after waking up in the middle of the night and going back to sleep. Again, the episodes take place at the moment of sleep onset. Occasionally, the jerking movements may be accompanied by a sensation of falling or other sensory symptoms.

Hypnic jerks may occur following a period of stress, fatigue, or sleep deprivation. The only treatment required is an explanation with reassurance.

81. I am having episodes where I cannot move one side of my entire body, arm, or leg at sleep onset or on awakening. These episodes last only a few minutes. I am frightened. Are these events forerunners of a sinister neurological illness?

A feeling of paralysis of an arm, leg, or the entire body at sleep onset or on awakening from sleep (sleep offset) is called **sleep paralysis**. Such episodes usually last for one to three minutes and disappear either sponta- neously or when someone touches the body. The per- son is usually conscious of the environment but feels very frightened and anxious.

Isolated sleep paralysis is a normal physiologic phe- nomenon experienced by many normal individuals without any associated disease. It also represents one of the clinical features of the narcolepsy syndrome (see Question 42). Isolated sleep paralysis may affect as many as 40 to 50 percent of individuals with normal sleep at least once during one's lifetime.

The first episode of sleep paralysis usually occurs in young adults and adolescents, and the condition affects both men and women. Episodes are triggered by sleep deprivation, stress, and shift work. Occasionally, isolated sleep paralysis runs in the family. Neurological examina- tion in persons experiencing isolated sleep paralysis will give normal results. If the affected individual has intense anxiety about the condition, however, he or she should

Sleep paralysis

Feeling of paralysis of limbs and/or body at sleep onset or awakening from sleep.

consult a family physician, who may refer the patient to a sleep specialist. In patients with sleep paralysis associated with narcolepsy, an overnight sleep recording during an episode shows loss of tone in the muscle recordings associated with waking brain electrical activity.

PART SEVEN

Sleep Disorders and Other Illnesses

82. I have difficulty getting to sleep and, many times, I wake up in the middle of the night. I am an anxious-type person and periodically become depressed. Can anxiety and depression cause sleep problems?

Anxiety and depression are the two most common psychiatric problems co-existing with sleep disturbance in the general population.

Obsessive-compulsive disorder

Condition characterized by repeated obsessions or intrusive thoughts and compulsions or repetitive compulsive behavior.

Anxiety and depression are the two most common psychiatric problems co-existing with sleep disturbance in the general population. Anxiety is the most common psychiatric illness, followed by depression. Anxiety disorders may include generalized anxiety disorder, phobia or fear, **obsessive-compulsive disorder (OCD)**, panic disorder, and post-traumatic stress disorder (PTSD). Insomnia is the most common sleep problem in patients with anxiety disorder. Patients present with difficulty getting to sleep and remaining asleep—they wake up repeatedly throughout the night, causing them to receive an inadequate amount of sleep.

OCD is characterized by repeated obsessions or intrusive thoughts and compulsions or repetitive compulsive behavior secondary to obsessions. In OCD patients, obsessions and compulsions are associated with severe anxiety and sleep disturbance.

Although most panic attacks occur during the daytime, some may arise during sleep. Affected individuals wake up at night with extreme fear and anxiety, palpitation, rapid heartbeat, heavy breathing, tremulousness, sweating, and fear of impending heart attacks or death. Panic attacks generally occur during the non-dream stage of sleep but sometimes may happen during the dream stage. Most patients with panic attacks complain of sleep maintenance and sleep initiation problems.

Patients with PTSD are prone to anxiety-provoking dreams and flashbacks. These episodes occur during REM sleep (dream stage) as well as NREM sleep (non-dream stage). Post-traumatic, life-threatening, or unpleasant events (for example, torture, war, Holocaust experiences, or other physical and sexual abuse in the past) are reenacted during the dreams of PTSD patients. They suffer from chronic insomnia and are in a hyperarousal state. Some investigators consider PTSD to be a disorder of REM sleep.

Anxiety and depression sometimes coexist. Several epidemiological surveys have clearly shown an association between insomnia and depression. In addition, studies have shown that individuals with insomnia are many times more likely to develop a new psychiatric disorder—in particular, major depression, within a year of the onset of insomnia and even within a year after the improvement of insomnia. Approximately 90 percent of patients with major depression or mood disorders suffer from insomnia and a smaller percentage of patients present with excessive daytime sleepiness. A characteristic mode of presentation in depression is early morning awakening, which is more intense in older persons than it is in younger individuals. Overnight sleep studies (see Question 37) in depressed individuals characteristically show early-onset dream stage (REM) sleep, mal-distribution of REM cycles, increased number of eye movements during REM sleep, decreased deeper stage of sleep, and shorter total sleep time. Individuals with bipolar depression (those with up-and-down mood swings) particularly young individuals with this disease may have excessive daytime sleepiness rather than insomnia.

Because depression and anxiety commonly co-exist with insomnia, it is important to watch for signs of depression. Whether depression and anxiety are causing insomnia rather than co-existing with insomnia is not clear. Therefore, in a recent National Institutes of Health consensus conference, it was suggested that the term should be comorbid insomnia, that is, insomnia comorbid with depression and anxiety. These symptoms of depression may include loss of interest in work and most activities, depressed feelings, a change in weight, sleep disturbance, reduced concentration, feelings of worthlessness, or suicidal thoughts. Immediate professional help should be sought if such symptoms are noted, as effective treatment is available. In many patients with co-existing insomnia and depression, insomnia complaints improve after adequate treatment of depression.

Lewis's comments:

I am a 70-year-old man suffering from insomnia for many years but the symptoms have become more pronounced in the last year. Falling asleep has not been my problem as I can fall asleep generally within 30 minutes but I repeatedly wake up in the middle of the night and in the early morning. I also have been snoring very loudly but do not have excessive daytime sleepiness. At the sleep center, the doctor thought I might have both sleep apnea and insomnia and therefore, the doctor ordered an overnight sleep study (see Question 37). The overnight sleep study was performed in January of this year which showed that I have severe sleep apnea (see Question 39). For treating sleep apnea, I was offered CPAP titration treatment (see Question 59), however, I could not tolerate any type of mask mostly due to the pressure but also due to some psychological factors. The doctor later told me that my sleep apnea is predominantly positional, that is, I either stop breathing or the breathing becomes ineffective when I am lying on my back but not when lying on the lateral positions. The doctor therefore advised me to practice sleeping on my side for my sleep apnea. My insomnia complaint persisted and I have been suffering also from depression and anxiety and the doctor thought that this was most likely related to the depression and I should consult a psychiatrist for appropriate antidepressant medications. My psychiatrist added Remeron to my other antidepressant medications. Following treatment with Remeron at bedtime my problem with middle of the night awakenings has improved considerably. Therefore, these medications, particularly the Remeron have improved my depression and insomnia symptoms. I also understand that it is important for me to sleep on my side and that I should not gain any weight. I will continue to see my sleep specialist in addition to my psychiatrist on a regular basis for monitoring my sleep apnea and insomnia.

83. I am a 30-year-old woman who has been suffering from depression for a long time. This depression is particularly notable during the winter; during the summer, I feel fine. I have terrible sleep problems during the winter. What can I do?

The symptoms described here are typical of seasonal affective depression (SAD), also known as winter depression. In this condition, symptoms of depression begin to appear in the months of October–November, when the hours of darkness (nighttime) begin to exceed the hours of light (daytime). The symptoms of depression gradually lift in the spring and summer as the days lengthen. In addition to depression in the winter, SAD-affected individuals have an excessive appetite with cravings for carbohydrates and weight gain. The condition is more common in younger women than in older women and more common in higher latitudes (northern climate).

Many SAD patients respond to bright light exposure in the morning. You should ask your family physician to refer you to a sleep specialist, who may suggest bright light treatment for you if he or she is satisfied that you have SAD.

84. Are sleep and physical illness related? In other words, do fever and other illnesses alter sleep and, if so, what is the mechanism involved?

A clear relationship exists between physical illness and sleep.

A clear relationship exists between physical illness and sleep. Sleep disruption is common in most medical and surgical conditions; sleep difficulty, in turn, affects these conditions adversely, interfering with the natural history and recovery process. The body's immune functions are negatively affected by sleep disruption. Consequently, our defense against infections caused by bacteria or viruses is impaired and it may take us longer to recover from disease. Sleep, therefore, may act as a host defense against disease by promoting immune functions and helping us recover from illness more rapidly. It should be noted, however, that the clinical consequences of sleep deprivation on immune function are very controversial.

85. My father has angina and heart failure. His sleep at night is very disturbed. Can it be due to heart problems?

Sleep disturbances in the form of difficulty in initiating sleep and maintaining sleep continuity are very common in a variety of medical disorders, including heart disease. Your father suffers from angina and heart failure, which often cause not only nighttime sleep disturbance but also excessive sleepiness in the daytime as a result of the disturbed and inadequate amount of sleep at night.

How does angina or heart failure cause sleep disturbance? **Angina** results from a narrowing of the coronary arteries (blood vessels supplying oxygen and metabolites to the heart). When angina patients exert themselves, there is a lack of blood supply to the heart relative to the demand. This imbalance causes chest pain. Sometimes the pain may awaken the patient at night—a condition known as nocturnal angina. Some patients wake up frequently at night, resulting in insufficient hours of sleep. Nocturnal angina may arise during both the dream and non-dream stages of sleep, but most often occurs during the dream stage of sleep. Many investigators have noted an association between sleep disturbances and anginal attacks. Some such patients also have sleep apnea (see Question 39), which causes reduced blood oxygen saturation and thus renders them more susceptible to anginal pain.

In some cases, patients may experience heart attacks as a result of inadequate blood supply to a particular portion of the muscle of the heart; a small area of the

Angina

Chest pain due to narrowing of coronary arteries, resulting in lack of blood supply to the heart relative to demand.

Many investigators have noted an association between sleep disturbances and anginal attacks.

141

muscle of the heart is then damaged, which in turn damages the heart muscle pump. These events may result in **heart failure** when the heart muscle cannot pump blood adequately to different body regions. The ensuing failure of many organs, including the liver, lungs, and brain, may result in shortness of breath, leg swelling, impairment of memory, difficulty sleeping at night, and excessive sleepiness in the daytime. Such patients need urgent attention from both heart and sleep specialists.

Adequate investigations and treatment for anginal pain and heart failure using drugs, oxygen inhalation, and sometimes special treatment for sleep apnea can improve the quality of life for such patients. In addition, they may prevent irregularities of heart rhythm and sudden death.

Heart failure

Inability of the heart to pump blood adequately to different body regions.

86. I have acid regurgitation, which wakes me up frequently at night, disturbing my sleep. What shall I do?

Acid regurgitation is a condition in which acid from the stomach flows back into the **esophagus** (the lower part of the food tube connected to the stomach) and into the mouth. The acid acts as an irritant, causing a burning sensation behind the breastbone (heartburn) and leaving a pungent, sour taste in the mouth. These symptoms frequently occur when a person is lying down in bed at night during sleep. The burning pain causes frequent awakenings, difficulty going back to sleep, and insufficient sleep. Such reflux disease is common in middle-aged and elderly people and sometimes in younger women during pregnancy.

Acid regurgitation

Condition in which acid from the stomach flows back into the esophagus.

Esophagus

Lower part of the food tube connected to the stomach.

142

The symptoms of acid reflux can be relieved by sitting up or by ingesting food or acid suppressant medications. Repeated episodes, causing inflammation of the lower esophagus, may lead to a condition that is a precursor to cancer of the esophagus. Consequently, medical advice regarding this condition should be sought early.

Sometimes acid reflux disease may cause aspiration of the stomach contents into the respiratory passages, giving rise to **aspiration pneumonia** (inflammation of the lungs). Nocturnal anginal pain (see Question 85) may also be mistaken for heartburn. Although anginal pain generally occurs on exertion, the particular variety called nocturnal angina may be difficult to differentiate from heartburn caused by reflux disease. Reflux heartburn is usually relieved by sitting up; in contrast, anginal pain is not necessarily relieved by taking such a position. When the pain travels to the neck, jaw, or left arm, anginal pain should be strongly suspected and urgent help should be sought.

Aspiration pneumonia

Inflammation of the lungs caused by aspiration of the stomach contents into the respiratory passages.

87. I have been excessively sleepy in the daytime. I wake up frequently at night. My doctor took a blood test and told me that I had low functioning of the thyroid gland. Can my excessive sleepiness be due to thyroid problems and, if so, can it be treated?

This problem may be caused by sleep apnea (see Question 39), which is sometimes associated with reduced function of the thyroid gland (located in front of the windpipe in the neck). Normal thyroid gland function is important for body metabolism. Reduced thyroid function commonly occurs in middle-aged and elderly individuals, and it is more common in women than men. The patient may complain of fatigue and constant tiredness, weight gain, slowing down physically and mentally, dryness of the skin, sensitivity to cold temperature, constipation, sometimes anginal pain, and sleep apnea. Cessation of breathing or marked reduction of breathing during sleep in this condition may reflect deposition of fatty tissues in the region of the upper airway passage, which obstructs airflow to the lungs during sleep. In addition, reduced function of the thyroid gland may affect regulation of the brain centers controlling respiration. Because of repeated apneas during sleep, the patient may wake up frequently at night, causing severe sleep disturbance. The insufficient sleep at night leads to excessive sleepiness in the daytime. This sleepiness could, of course, be related to the reduced function of the thyroid gland alone, without associated sleep apnea.

Reduced function of the thyroid gland can be effectively treated with thyroid replacement medication.

Reduced function of the thyroid gland can be effectively treated with thyroid replacement medication. Some patients may also need a special mask treatment for sleep apnea (see Question 59). Reports in the literature suggest that adequate treatment of sleep apnea can completely relieve sleep disturbance, daytime sleepiness, and other symptoms resulting from reduced thyroid function. If you have such symptoms, it is imperative to consult your family physician and a sleep specialist early to avoid any serious long-term complications.

88. I always feel tired and fatigued. I also suffer from aches and pains all over my body and certain spots are tender to touch. I have difficulty sleeping. My friend has heard of conditions called fibromyalgia and chronic fatigue syndrome. Is it possible that I have fibromyalgia or chronic fatigue syndrome, and do these conditions cause sleep disturbance?

Fibromyalgia

Type of rheumatoid disease that does not affect bones or joints.

Chronic fatigue syndrome

Condition characterized by feelings of profound fatigue and functioning below the usual level of energy which is not improved by bed rest.

Both **fibromyalgia** and **chronic fatigue syndrome** can cause nighttime sleep disturbance, daytime fatigue, tiredness, and sleepiness. An estimated 3 to 6 million Americans suffer from fibromyalgia, a type of rheumatoid disease that does not affect bones or joints. Individuals suffering from this condition complain of diffuse muscle aches and pains throughout the body but most commonly in the neck, shoulders, lower back, and buttocks. No single diagnostic laboratory test can detect fibromyalgia. Instead, the condition is diagnosed based on history and physical examination, and after exclusion of other causes of muscle, bone, and joint pains. The cause of fibromyalgia remains undetermined, but many researchers are studying it in order to better understand the nature of the illness.

An estimated 3 to 6 million Americans suffer from fibromyalgia, a type of rheumatoid disease that does not affect bones or joints.

Sleep complaint is very common with fibromyalgia. Patients complain of repeated awakenings and decreased amount of total sleep. Sleep is not restorative or refreshing. As a result of the nighttime sleep disturbance, patients complain of daytime fatigue and sleepiness. An overnight sleep study (see Question 37) may show intrusion of waking brain electrical activity into the sleep pattern, though the same findings have been noted in several other conditions and even in some normal people. Some patients with fibromyalgia experience repeated leg jerking during sleep at night (see Question 45), which could be documented during an overnight sleep study. Sleep specialists recommend a combination of treatments for fibromyalgia: drug therapy with tricyclic antidepressants; short-term use of sleeping medications; an exercise program; education; and reassurance. Recently the Food and Drug Administration (FDA) approved pregabalin (lyrica), a centrally acting drug used to treat neuropathic pain and adults with partial epitepsy, of the management of fibromyalgia.

Fibromyalgia and chronic fatigue syndrome (CFS) share some overlapping symptoms. Both conditions remain controversial and have undetermined causes. Many patients with CFS report nighttime sleep disturbance, daytime fatigue and sleepiness, similar to the symptoms noted in fibromyalgia patients. An overnight sleep study may show delayed sleep onset and repeated awakenings in CFS patients, but no such study has been performed in a large number of patients. Both fibromyalgia and CFS may have comorbid sleep disorders such as sleep apnea, RLS and PLMS.

CFS is a complex and debilitating illness. Patients complain of profound fatigue, functioning below their usual level of energy, which is not improved by bed rest. CFS affects more than one million people in the United States and is more common in women than men. An international panel of experts established the diagnostic criteria for CFS (see **Table 9**). Diagnosis of CFS depends on the patient's history and the information gathered via physical examination, as well as exclusion of other causes for the fatigue after extensive laboratory investigations. Some patients with CFS

CFS affects more than one million people in the United States and is more common in women than men.

146

Table 9 Diagnostic Criteria for Chronic Fatigue Syndrome

- Severe chronic fatigue for 6 months or longer
- Absence of other medical conditions explaining chronic fatigue
- Presence of 4 or more of the following features:
  - Impairment of short-term memory or concentration
  - Sore throat
  - Tender lymph nodes
  - Muscle pain
  - Multiple joint pain without swelling or tenderness
  - Headache different from any previous headache
  - Unrefreshing sleep
  - Post-exertional malaise lasting longer than 24 hours

may have depression or other psychological problems. Over the years, investigators have suggested a variety of viruses as possible causes of this disease, but as yet none has been definitely associated with the condition.

One important laboratory test in diagnosis of CFS is recording of blood pressure and pulse rate on a tilt table, because many patients show a fall of blood pressure in the upright position, which causes fainting feelings. In such patients, drugs can be used to maintain the blood pressure while they are standing. In other patients, treatment is similar to that suggested for fibromyalgia.

89. I suffer from emphysema and chronic bronchitis. I have been experiencing sleep problems lately. Can my sleep problems be due to my lung disease?

Lung disease is an important medical cause of sleep problems. Patients with chronic **bronchitis** (inflammation of the lower airway passage) and **emphysema** (excessive stretching of the lungs) suffer from chronic cough, shortness of breath on exertion, and tightness

Bronchitis

Inflammation of the lower airway passage.

Emphysema

Excessive stretching of the lungs.

Lung disease is an important medical cause of sleep problems.

147

in the chest. Listening to the chest with a stethoscope reveals many abnormalities, particularly during an acute episode, which can be confirmed by chest X-rays and lung function tests in the laboratory.

During breathing, air exchange occurs in the lungs to maintain normal blood oxygen levels. Because of the disease affecting the lungs and the lower airways, air exchange is impaired. As a result, blood oxygen levels fall below the normal range and decline even further during sleep at night. Many patients who suffer from chronic bronchitis and long-term emphysema develop chronic heart failure and irregular heart rhythm. In these individuals, sleep disturbance may include difficulty getting to sleep and repeated awakenings throughout the night, causing insufficient sleep and daytime sleepiness. Other factors which may contribute to sleep disturbance in such patients include medications used to treat emphysema and chronic bronchitis, and increased cough due to excessive accumulation of secretions in the **bronchi** (airway passages to the lungs). Sometimes, the condition may coexist with sleep apnea.

Chronic bronchitis and emphysema are serious conditions. It is advisable to consult both lung and sleep specialists so that appropriate tests may be performed to diagnose and institute optimal treatment.

Bronchi

Airway passages to the lungs.

Chronic bronchitis and emphysema are serious conditions.

90. I suffer from allergy and bronchial asthma. Can these conditions be responsible for my sleep difficulty?

Bronchial asthma causes a variety of sleep disturbances including early morning awakenings, difficulty maintaining sleep and excessive daytime sleepiness similar to those noted in patients with emphysema and chronic bronchitis. Patients with bronchial asthma suffer from intermittent episodes of respiratory distress, wheezing, and cough. Prolonged episodes lasting for hours could be life-threatening. Asthma attacks may occur at any hour of the day or night, and worsening of the symptoms at night is a frequent observation in such patients as a result of progressive constriction of the lower airway passages (bronchi) to the lungs. Coexisting sleep apnea is present in many affected individuals. Patients should consult both lung and sleep specialists for adequate investigations and treatment of their condition.

91. I have Lyme disease. Can it cause sleep disturbances?

Although sleep complaints are common in Lyme disease, adequate studies in a large number of patients have not been conducted to fully elucidate the link between sleeping problems and this condition. Patients may experience difficulty going to sleep at night, wake up repeatedly during sleep, have insufficient hours of sleep, and suffer from daytime fatigue and sleepiness.

Lyme disease is caused by infection with an organism that is transmitted to humans by tick bites. Shortly after the tick bite, the infected individual develops a characteristic skin rash, followed by fever, general malaise, and tiredness. Weeks to months after the initial illness, approximately 60 percent of patients will develop joint problems; in 8 to 15 percent, the nervous system and the heart may be affected. Professional help should be sought at the slightest suspicion during the initial period, because the disease shows an excel-

Lyme disease
infection caused by an organism transmitted to humans by tick bites.

lent response to treatment with antibiotics shortly after the onset of illness following tick bites.

92. I had paralytic poliomyelitis as a young adult and made a reasonably good recovery from my paralysis. Now at the age of 60, I am again experiencing weakness of my previously paralyzed leg and am also feeling some weakness in other extremities. In addition, I have aches and pains and sleep problems. Am I developing postpolio syndrome?

Postpolio syndrome

Weakness of arm or leg formerly affected by poliomyelitis, accompanied by paralysis of muscles including those of the previously unaffected extremities, and often breathing difficulties.

Poliomyelitis

Inflammation of the spinal cord, often called Infantile Paralysis.

You may have **postpolio syndrome**. With this syndrome, there is usually a history of **poliomyelitis** in childhood or early adult life, accompanied by paralysis of muscles and often breathing difficulties. Years after recovering from the initial illness, the patient may visit a physician with complaints of weakness of the previously affected arm or leg plus weakness of the muscles of the other extremities. Patients also complain of aches and pains and sleep difficulty. The sleep problems may reflect the past involvement of the nerve cells in the brain which control sleep-wake systems and breathing centers. Whether there is further involvement of the nerve cells years later remains unknown; the exact mechanism of postpolio syndrome has not yet been elucidated.

Many such patients have sleep apnea (see Question 39), which can be documented only by an overnight sleep study (see Question 37). As a result of repeated apneas and reduced ventilation during sleep, they may wake up frequently, causing interrupted sleep and excessive daytime sleepiness. It is important to diagnose the nature of the sleep and breathing abnormalities, because effective treatment is available. Without treatment, patients may develop long-term adverse consequences associated with sleep-related breathing disturbances (see Question 39).

93. My friend suffers from Lou Gehrig's disease. He is having lots of sleep and breathing difficulties. Should he see a sleep specialist?

Your friend should definitely see a sleep specialist. **Lou Gehrig's disease** (amyotrophic lateral sclerosis or ALS) is a serious condition characterized by progressive death of the nerve cells controlling muscles of the body. An affected individual also suffers loss of function of the nerve cells regulating breathing. As a result, he or she develops breathing difficulties, which worsen during sleep—giving rise to sleep apnea (see Question 39) and lowering of blood oxygen saturation. Sleep difficulties result from repeated episodes of apnea during sleep. Sleep is profoundly disturbed, and the patient has excessive daytime sleepiness.

Although no treatment can halt the progression of ALS, the patient's quality of life may be considerably improved by treating the sleeping and breathing difficulties. Measures are available to assist ventilation, which will improve breathing and sleep, and hence enhance daytime function and these measures will also prevent repeated hospitalizations. Whether such measurers will alter the natural history of the illness,

Lou Gehrig's disease

Amyotrophic lateral sclerosis (ALS). A serious condition characterized by progressive death of nerve cells controlling muscles of the body.

which, is a gradual progression, can not be definitely stated, but there are indications from some studies that such treatment of respiratory failure using intermittent positive airway pressure ventilation may prolong life and definitely improve the quality of life of ALS patients, and, therefore, secondarily improve the sleep function of the caregivers. It is, therefore, important to seek help from a sleep specialist in addition to consulting with a neurologist and a lung specialist.

94. I have been told that stroke may cause sleep disorder and sleep apnea. Is this true?

Many patients with stroke complain of sleep disruption and sleep complaints, resulting from sleep apnea and other causes. Some report insomnia with repeated awakenings during sleep at night due to associated depression; others experience muscle stiffness and paralysis, which makes it difficult for the individuals to move.

An increasing body of evidence, taken from several surveys and laboratory studies, indicates that sleep apnea and stroke are intimately related.

An increasing body of evidence, taken from several surveys and laboratory studies, indicates that sleep apnea and stroke are intimately related. Sleep apnea may render an individual more susceptible to developing stroke, and stroke itself may make the person more susceptible to sleep apnea. Stroke and sleep apnea share some common risk factors, which should be kept in mind for preventive treatment. These risk factors include high blood pressure, heart disease, older age, obesity, smoking, and alcohol consumption.

Sleep apnea may adversely affect the long-term outcome in patients with stroke. It is important to make such a diagnosis early because effective treatment is available for the sleep disorder, which may also decrease the risk of future stroke.

95. I am a diabetic and am experiencing tingling and numbness in my legs. My doctor told me that I have nerve disease related to uncontrollable diabetes mellitus. Can this condition be responsible for my disturbed sleep?

Your disturbed sleep may very definitely result from nerve disease related to diabetes mellitus. Long-standing diabetes mellitus is the most common cause of disease of the nerves innervating the extremities, head, neck, and trunk. The probability of involvement of the nerves increases when the diabetes is not well controlled. Affected patients may complain of tingling and numbness, most commonly initially in the legs; advanced cases may involve the arms and other parts of the body. In addition to sensory complaints, patients may have weakness and wasting of the muscles, particularly those in the legs below the knees bilaterally. Often, they complain of burning pain in the legs. In addition, nerves supplying the muscles of respiration may be affected, causing breathing problems that become worse during sleep.

Long-standing diabetes mellitus is the most common cause of disease of the nerves innervating the extremities, head, neck, and trunk.

Sleep disturbances in diabetic **neuropathy** (nerve involvement) are caused by a combination of factors: pain associated with the nerve disease and immobility due to severe weakness of the muscles may cause difficulty getting to sleep and repeated awakenings. Sleep-related breathing difficulties, such as cessation of

Neuropathy
Risk factor for RLS involving affection of peripheral nerves.

breathing or marked reduction of the volume of air inhaled during sleep, will reduce the blood oxygen saturation and cause repeated awakenings, disturbing sleep. Because of the nighttime sleep disturbance, the patient may complain of excessive sleepiness during the daytime.

It is important to strictly follow the advice of a physician to keep diabetes under control so as to avoid the long-term complications of diabetic neuropathy.

96. I have Parkinson's disease and am taking medications for this condition. Lately, I have been experiencing sleep difficulties. Can my sleep problem be due to Parkinson's disease or the medications used to treat Parkinson's disease?

Parkinson's disease (PD)

A degenerative disorder of the central nervous system that often impairs the sufferer's motor skills and speech.

Sleep problems in PD can be caused by the disease itself or by the medications used to treat this disease.

Investigators who have studied sleep problems in **Parkinson's disease** (PD) estimate that 70 to 90 percent of patients complain of sleep difficulties. These sleep problems include insomnia, excessive daytime sleepiness, abnormal movements or behavior during sleep, and, in some patients, inability to go to sleep at the right time.

Sleep problems in PD can be caused by the disease itself or by the medications used to treat this disease. Inability to turn over during the night, inability to get out of bed without help, cramps or jerks in the legs, muscle stiffness, back pain, and a desire to urinate frequently at night are some of the factors disturbing sleep in these patients. Patients may also complain of excessive daytime sleepiness, abnormal movements and noise making during the dream stage of sleep, and disturbing dreams. Some individuals may have sleep apnea with repeated awakenings and disruption of sleep. Sleep problems are more common in the advanced stage of the disease. PD patients also have an increased prevalence of depression, which may cause sleep abnormalities.

Some PD patients observe a "sleep benefit." On first waking up in the morning, they may note an improvement in muscle stiffness and tremor, both of which are common and disabling manifestations of PD. This improvement lasts, on average, an hour and a half; the underlying mechanism is not definitely known.

Medications used to treat PD may also have adverse effects on sleep. In particular, the medications may give rise to abnormal movements and vivid or frightening dreams or hallucinations, which disrupt sleep by causing repeated awakenings and arousals. Both the medications used to treat PD and the disease itself may be responsible for irresistible sleep attacks and excessive daytime sleepiness in some patients.

Treatment of PD does not consistently improve sleep in these patients. Some researchers report improvements in both sleep and the symptoms of PD with therapy; other reports indicate that sleep abnormalities persist. An adjustment of the dose, an additional bedtime dose of an antiparkinsonian medication, or administration of a longer-acting preparation of an antiparkinsonian medication may sometimes alleviate the PD symptoms, though they may reappear later. Sometimes, a second dose of medication may be needed in the middle of the night, and this may help

patients with insomnia. One should be careful, however, because increasing the dose of antiparkinsonian
medications may cause hallucinations and vivid
dreams, disturbing sleep. If patients suffer from abnormal movements and behavior during the dream stage
of sleep, rapid eye movement behavior disorder (see
Question 46) should be suspected. With this condition, a small dose of benzodiazepines at bedtime will
be helpful. Effective treatments are also available for
hallucinations and psychotic episodes occurring at
night. In those patients with repeated episodes of sleep
apneas, treatment via a mask (see Question 59) may
prove helpful.

Listen to the comments made by Orhan, a 69-year-old
patient with Parkinson's Disease and sleep apnea:

*I was first diagnosed with Parkinson's Disease in early
1997 and actually started taking medication for Parkinson's Disease in 1999. During this period, my sleep pattern
has become very much fragmented believed to be due to
Parkinson's Disease. My wife was also complaining that I
was snoring loudly at night and I was also frequently
falling asleep for short periods throughout the day. I was
then referred to a sleep specialist who after taking my history and physical examination ordered an overnight
polysomnographic study (see Question 37), multiple sleep
latency tests (MSLT; see Question 38) following the overnight study and actigraphy (see Question 36). My overnight stay at the sleep center was a pleasant experience in a
comfortable room under the care of an efficient and professional technologist who explained the procedure to me and
placed various sensors on my head and body recording
brain waves, breathing patterns, snoring, blood oxygen*

saturation, body movements and muscle activities. Follow-ing the overnight sleep study, I had MSLT test performed in the daytime for 4 studies at intervals of 2 hours and each time lasting for 20 minutes. The sleep specialist then reviewed all my tests and reported that I had a severe upper airway obstructive sleep apnea (see Question 39), which caused me to stop breathing or have ineffective breathing repeatedly throughout the night associated with reduced blood oxygen saturation, recurrent awakenings and broken sleep patterns. The daytime study showed that I went to sleep very quickly. My actigraphy study (see Ques-tion 36) documented an average of 4 hours of sleep at night and even that short sleep was fragmented due to repeated movements and awakenings. The doctor suggested CPAP titration treatment (see Question 59) for me. An addi-tional overnight monitoring at the sleep center was needed to select the proper pressure, mask size and type. Based on trials and personal choice for comfort, a nasal pillow type mask was selected for using with the CPAP machine. I have been using this equipment every night during sleep for a year now. My sleep has improved immensely and I do not fall asleep in the daytime and I do not snore (according to my wife) since I started my CPAP, thanks to the special-ist at the sleep center.

97. My father, who is 71, suffers from Alzheimer's disease. At night, he is agitated and screams and shouts later at night. Is this problem due to Alzheimer's disease, related dementia or is he developing another disorder?

Alzheimer's disease is the most common cause of dementia in middle-aged to elderly individuals account-ing for at least 60% cases of chronic dementia. It is

Alzheimer's disease is the most common cause of dementia in middle-aged to elderly individuals accounting for at least 60% cases of chronic dementia.

characterized by progressive intellectual deterioration. Patients may develop agitation, hallucination, and confusion, which become worse at night. Many affected individuals suffer from severe sleep disturbances in the advanced stage of the illness.

In the patient described in the question, the nighttime agitation, screaming, and shouting most likely are related to the advanced stage of Alzheimer's disease. Many patients with this condition suffer from **"sundowning,"** which is characterized by episodes of nocturnal confusion associated with partial or complete inversion of sleep rhythms, that is, increased wakefulness at night and sleepiness in the daytime. When the lights are turned off at night, the patient becomes fearful and agitated, and begins to scream and shout. For many of these patients, use of a night lamp may prove helpful.

Sundowning

Nocturnal confusion associated with partial or complete inversion of sleep rhythms.

Sleep dysfunction in Alzheimer's disease may occur even in the early stages,, but is more common and severe in the advanced stages of the illness. In addition to sundowning, these patients often sleep early in the evening, waking up frequently and stay up most of the night. As a result of this broken or fragmented sleep, they have excessive daytime sleepiness. The sleep disturbance causing insomnia and daytime sleepiness (inversion of sleep rhythm) may reflect the involvement of the nerve cells controlling sleep/wake regulation and sleep rhythms.

Other factors linked to sleep disorders in Alzheimer's disease patients include associated depression and periodic jerking movements of the legs (periodic limb movements in sleep; see Question 45). Depression is common in elderly subjects without dementia, however, and may cause sleep disturbance which is different from the sleep dysfunction noted in patients with Alzheimer's dementia. Overnight sleep recording (see Question 37) shows a characteristic pattern of early-onset dream stage of sleep and an increased number of rapid eye movements at this stage of sleep in patients with depression. These findings are quite different from the reduced rapid eye movements and reduced amount of dream stage sleep in patients in the advanced stages of Alzheimer's disease.

Another important cause of nighttime sleep disturbance in patients with Alzheimer's disease is sleep apnea, which affects 33 to 53 percent of such individuals. Some controversy persists regarding whether sleep apnea increases with severity of the illness or its rapid progression. Sleep apnea may, of course, lower the blood oxygen levels, which in turn may cause nighttime confusion and agitation.

Another important cause of nighttime sleep disturbance in patients with Alzheimer's disease is sleep apnea, which affects 33 to 53 percent of such individuals.

Other causes of sleep disturbances in patients with Alzheimer's disease may include medications that the patients have been taking and associated general medical disorders, such as heart disease or lung disease.

98. My cousin, aged 30, has been suffering from a muscle disorder since the age of 20. Now, he is always sleeping in the daytime. Can muscle disease cause sleep problems?

Muscle diseases can cause sleep problems, primarily through sleep-related breathing disorders. Although muscle diseases may be inherited, sometimes they occur without any family history. Patients complain of weakness and wasting of the muscles in the upper arms and upper legs, causing difficulty in walking, getting up from a sitting position, and raising the arms above the shoulders. Such diseases may also strike the muscles that control breathing.

Affected patients present with excessive sleepiness in the daytime as a result of repeated arousals during nighttime sleep. Because of the involvement of the muscles controlling their breathing, they stop breathing repeatedly throughout the night or their breathing is markedly reduced. As a consequence, the blood oxygen saturation level decreases and the patients repeatedly wake up throughout the night.

In such cases, it is important to direct attention to the possibility of sleep-related breathing disturbances. Strong clues include excessive daytime sleepiness, breathlessness during the waking period and unexplained edema (swelling of the legs due to collection of fluid under the skin) for which no apparent cause is found. An overnight sleep study (see Question 37) will detect the sleep-related breathing disturbances and any fall of blood oxygen levels during sleep. It is important to diagnose these problems, because effective treatment is available—for example, assisted ventilation and breathing through a mask. Treatment can alleviate the sleep problems; prevent long-term complications such as heart failure, irregular heart rhythms, and intellectual deterioration; and improve the quality of life to a considerable extent.

99. My mother has been diagnosed with depression and takes a variety of medications. She is always falling asleep in the daytime. Can these medications cause sleep problems?

Side effects may occur with all medications including antidepressants.

A variety of antidepressants and mood stabilizers are used to treat patients with depression. Side effects may occur with all medications, including antidepressants. Some of these medications have a prolonged elimination time and, hence, persisting effects in the daytime, causing sedation and sleepiness in the daytime. Side effects vary depending on the class of medications (e.g., tricyclics [TCA]; selective serotonin reuptake inhibitors [SSRI]; monoamine oxidase [MAO] inhibitors; drugs with "other" mechanisms; and mood stabilizers). Some antidepressants (for example amitriptyline, trazodone) have hypnotic properties. These drugs are generally recommended for evening use. If they are used during the daytime, they will cause the patient to fall asleep in the daytime.

Most antidepressants belonging to the **tricyclic group** (so named because these drugs have a 3-ring chemical structure) and some drugs belonging to other classes will cause daytime sleepiness and impairment of function during the daytime.

Tricyclic group
Drugs having a 3-ring chemical structure.

Other drugs such as Prozac and Lithium may have alerting effects, disturbing nighttime sleep with repeated awakenings and exerting some sedative effects during the daytime.

In addition to the potential for antidepressant medications to cause excessive daytime sleepiness, the depression itself may cause excessive sleepiness.

You should consult your physician before discontinuing medications because of excessive sleepiness and other side effects because abrupt withdrawal, rather than gradual tapering, may cause discontinuation syndrome (e.g., withdrawal, rebound and recurrence). Your doctor will be in the best position to either switch you to another drug, change the timing of the medication or gradually taper the medication off.

100. Does menopause interfere with sleep and, if so, how and why?

The hormonal disturbances present during menopause cause a variety of problems.

Menopausal symptoms include insomnia, hot flashes, and depression—mainly caused by the reduced amount of estrogen.

The hormonal disturbances present during menopause cause a variety of problems. In particular, estrogen and progesterone levels are reduced. The 2007 NSF Sleep in America poll found that 61% of post-menopausal women experience some symptoms of insomnia at least a few nights a week and 22% of these post-menopausal women have a difficult time sleeping due to hot flashes or night sweats. Symptoms of RLS also appear more frequently in these individuals than in other segments of the population. Menopausal symptoms include insomnia, hot flashes, and depression—mainly caused by the reduced amount of estrogen. Approximately 75 percent of women experience hot flashes during menopause; these events may be accompanied by excessive sweating, anxiety, and palpitation. Such symptoms may cause repeated awakenings during sleep. As a result, the menopausal woman's sleep is not consolidated, causing daytime fatigue and sleepiness. Sleep disturbance in menopausal women may partly be age-related (see Question 11). Because the symptoms improve on estrogen treatment, however, estrogen is likely the main factor involved.

Sleep problems in menopausal women may also follow from sleep-disordered breathing problems. The prevalence of sleep apnea in pre-menopausal women is much lower than that in men; after menopause, however, the prevalence in women approaches that in men. The issue of whether sleep apnea is related to estrogen deficiency remains controversial.

Resources

You can obtain essential information about sleep and sleep disorders from a number of professional and lay organizations. A number of Web sites also disseminate valuable information about sleep and sleep disorders directed specifically to the public; this information has been written by doctors. In addition, many books are devoted to sleep medicine. The sources listed here should point you in the right direction.

American Academy of Sleep Medicine (AASM)
One Westbrook Corporate Center, Suite 920
Westchester, IL 60154
Telephone: 708-492-0930
www.aasm.org
The mission of the AASM is to promote sleep disorders medicine to members of the medical and paramedical professions as well as to the public. The organization is dedicated to supporting quality care for patients with sleep disorders, providing professional and public education on the issues, and encouraging and supporting research in sleep medicine.

American Sleep Apnea Association (ASAA)
1424 K Street NW, Suite 302
Washington, DC 20005
Telephone 202-293-3650
www.sleepapnea.org
The ASAA is devoted to helping patients with sleep apnea and works with a variety of support groups in the United States.

Narcolepsy Network (NN)
79A Main Street
North Kingstown, RI 02852
Toll Free Telephone 888-292-4522
www.narcolepsynetwork.org
The NN disseminates educational material on narcolepsy and
helps develop narcolepsy support groups.

National Center for Sleep Disorders Research (NCSDR)
2 Rockledge Center, Suite 7024
6701 Rockledge Drive, MSC7920
Bethesda, MD 20892-7920
Telephone 301-435-0199
www.nhlbi.nih.gov/sleep
The NCSDR was established after a national commission on
sleep disorders research, which was mandated by Congress,
recommended in 1993 that a national center for research and
education in sleep and sleep disorders be established. This center is located within the National Heart, Lung, and Blood
Institute of the National Institutes of Health (NIH) in
Bethesda, Maryland. It supports research, education, and train-
ing in sleep and sleep disorders for all health care professionals.
The center also participates in public awareness and education
campaigns about sleep disorders. It works in collaboration with
several federal agencies, including the NIH, the former Alcohol, Drug Abuse, and Mental Health Administration, and the
Departments of Defense, Transportation, and Veterans Affairs.

National Sleep Foundation (NSF)
729 Fifteenth Street, NW, 4th Floor
Washington, DC 20005
Telephone 202-347-3471
The NSF produces valuable brochures dealing with sleep and
sleep disorders, promotes public education (particularly about
driving, fatigue, and sleepiness as well as important sleep disorders), and periodically organizes Gallup polls dealing with sleep
and sleep difficulties.

Restless Legs Syndrome (RLS) Foundation
1610 14th Street NW, Suite 300
Rochester, MN 55901
Telephone 507-287-6465
www.rls.org

The RLS Foundation was established by patients suffering from RLS in 1990 and is guided by an RLS scientific advisory board and a medical advisory board. Its mission is to support patients with RLS and their families. The RLS Foundation also provides information to educate health care providers about RLS and sponsors research intended to find better treatments and, eventually, a definitive cure. Members (patients with RLS) receive newsletters with valuable information about the disease and support groups throughout the country.

World Association of Sleep Medicine (WASM)
WASM Administrative Secretary
Klinikstr.16
Kassel D-34128
Germany
Fax: 49-561-6009-126
E-mail: WASMsecretary@gmx.de
Web site: www.wasmonline.org
The fundamental mission of the WASM is to advance sleep health worldwide. WASM will fulfill its mission by promoting and encouraging education, research and patient care throughout the world. WASM strives to advance knowledge about sleep and its disorders amongst both healthcare workers and the general public. WASM provides a forum for discussion and consideration of issues of relevance to particular regions and cultures. WASM has an online newsletter and the first issue deals with "Sleep Medicine Worldwide."

Recommended Books
1. Chokroverty S(ed). Sleep Disorders Medicine: Basic Science, Technical Considerations and Clinical Aspecs. Philidelphia, PA, USA, Elsevier/Butterworth
2. Chokroverty S. Clinical Companion to Sleep Disorders Medicine. Boston, MA, USA, Butterworth/Elsevier
3. Kryger MH, Roth T, Dement WC (eds). Principles and Practice of Sleep Medicine. Philidelphia, PA, USA, Elsevier/Saunders
4. Lee-Chiong TL (ed). Sleep: A Comprehensive Handbook. Hoboken, NJ, USA, Wiley-Liss.
5. Silber MH, Krahn LE, Morgenthaler QI (eds). Sleep Medicine in Clinical Practice. Boca Raton, FL, USA, Taylor and Francis

Glossary

Acetylcholine: The main chemical agent causing activation of REM sleep.

Acid regurgitation: Condition in which acid from the stomach flows back into the esophagus.

Actigraphy: Test involving wearing a watch-like device on the wrist or ankle to monitor activities of the body resulting from body movements.

Adenoids: Lymphoid tissues in the throat behind the nasal passage.

Angina: Chest pain due to narrowing of coronary arteries, resulting in lack of blood supply to the heart relative to demand.

Aspiration pneumonia: Inflammation of the lungs caused by aspiration of the stomach contents into the respiratory passages.

Augmentation: is characterized by intensification of RLS symptoms, occurring earlier than the initial period and spreading to other parts of the body. It is an adverse effect of dopaminergic medication noted mostly with Levodopa treatment.

Autonomic nervous system: the part of the nervous system controlling vital functions of the body such as circulation, respiration and hormone secretion.

Bariatric surgery: Procedure performed to assist obese patients in achieving weight loss.

Beta blockers: Class of drugs used to treat high blood pressure and heart disease.

Biphasic pattern: Sleep pattern observed especially in the elderly wherein napping during the daytime offsets a person's shorter nighttime sleep periods.

Brain stem: Deeper part in the base of the brain which connects the main brain hemisphere with the spinal cord.

Bronchi: Airway passages to the lungs.

Bronchitis: Inflammation of the lower airway passage.

Bruxism: Vigorous contraction of muscles of the upper jaw, which rubs the upper and lower teeth against each other.

Bulimia: Eating disorder characterized by cravings for excessive eating and drinking, followed by purging and vomiting.

Cataplexy: Momentary loss of muscle tone without loss of consciousness.

Cerebellum: Structure located below the main brain hemisphere which controls movements and coordination.

Cerebrospinal fluid: Fluid bathing the central nervous system.

Chronic fatigue syndrome: Condition characterized by feelings of profound fatigue and functioning below the usual level of energy which is not improved by bed rest.

Circadian rhythm: The daily pattern of human sleep-wake periods based on the Latin *circa* (about) and *dies* (day).

Cognitive behavioral therapy: Method of addressing dysfunctional beliefs and attitudes about sleep combined with other non-pharmacologic measures.

Confusional arousals: Episodes which may occur during deep dreamless sleep involving complex behaviors without conscious awareness.

Continuous positive airway pressure (CPAP): Remedial therapy involving a small portable machine used to deliver air through the nose to the back of the throat.

Comorbid: Pertaining to two or more disorders simultaneously.

CPAP device: A CPAP device includes a mask, head straps, tubes, and a fan. It reduces snoring and prevents apnea disturbances.

CPAP titration: Gradually adjusting the flow of air until the desired effect is achieved.

Decrement: To subtract or reduce, as observed in certain chemicals during sleep deprivation.

Delayed sleep phase syndrome (DSPS): Condition in which the major sleep episode is delayed relative to the desired clock time.

Diaphragm: Main muscle of breathing, located at the junction of the chest and abdomen.

Dopamine agonist: Compound that activates dopamine receptors.

Dopamine: Chemical which is deficient in patients with Parkinson's disease.

Dopaminergic medication: Agent promoting dopamine function.

Electroencephalogram (EEG): Recording of the electrical activities of the brain.

Electromyogram (EMG): Recording of the electrical activities of the muscles.

Electro-oculogram (EOG): Recording of the movements of the eye.

Emphysema: Excessive stretching of the lungs.

Epworth Sleepiness Scale: Tool used during diagnostic process to assess subjective evidence of sleepiness.

Esophagus: Lower part of the food tube connected to the stomach.

Etiology: Cause of a symptom or condition.

Expiration: Exhaling air during breathing.

Fibromyalgia: Type of rheumatoid disease that does not affect bones or joints.

Gamma-aminobutyric acid (GABA): Neurotransmitter that plays an important role in regulating REM as well as NREM sleep.

Glaucoma: Eye condition causing increased pressure within the eye, which may lead to blindness if left untreated.

Heart failure: Inability of the heart to pump blood adequately to different body regions.

Hemoglobin: Blood pigment, the color of which indicates blood oxygen saturation.

Histamine: One of the chemicals responsible for inactivation of REM sleep.

Homeostasis: Maintenance of internal equilibrium which ensures that a period of wakefulness is followed by a sleep debt and a propensity to sleep.

Hyperalgesia: Excessive perception of pain.

Hypersomnia: Recurrent episodes of excessive daytime sleepiness or prolonged nighttime sleep.

Hypnic jerks: Sudden jerking motions of the legs or whole body occurring at the moment of falling asleep.

Hypocretin 1: Peptide thought to be important in regulating the sleep/wake cycle.

Hypopnea: Reduction of breathing volume to below the normal level.

Hypothalamus: Center of control for secretion of hormones, food and water intake, body temperature, emotion and sleep-wake regulation.

Idiopathic: Not associated with other disease and no causes found.

Increment: To increase or add, as observed in certain chemicals during sleep deprivation.

Jet lag syndrome: Condition caused by travel outside one's own time zone in which the body's internal clock becomes out of synch with the external clock in a new time zone.

Kidneys: Organs responsible for urine production and excretion from the body.

Larks: Group of people, called morning types, who go to sleep early in the evening and wake up early in the morning.

Lewy Body disease: Chronic degenerative neurological illness resembling Parkinson's disease with dementia.

Lou Gehrig's disease: Amyotrophic lateral sclerosis (ALS). A serious condition characterized by progressive death of nerve cells controlling muscles of the body.

Lyme disease: infection caused by an organism transmitted to humans by tick bites.

Malocclusion: Condition in which the upper and lower teeth do not fit well.

Medulla: Part of the brain below the brain hemisphere controlling vital functions such as respiration, heart and circulation.

Melatonin: The hormone secreted by the pineal gland thought to help adjust our internal and external clocks.

Microsleep: Transient periods of NREM stage 1 sleep occuring during sleep deprivation experiments.

Micturition: Function of urination, increased frequency of which interferes with sleep.

Monophasic sleep pattern: Consolidated sleep at night only, as opposed to biphasic sleep pattern of two periods of sleep at night and a short nap in the daytime or polyphasic sleep pattern of several short periods of sleep throughout 24 hours as in newborn.

Multiple sleep latency (MSLT): Scoring system used to determine objective evidence of sleepiness.

Multiple sleep latency (MSLT): Test used to assess the severity of daytime sleepiness.

Multiple system atrophy: Chronic degenerative disease of the nervous system associated with features of Parkinson's disease.

Narcolepsy: A disorder of excessive sleepiness characterized by a marked reduction of a group of special nerve cells containing certain peptide chemicals.

Narcolepsy: Sleep disorder characterized by excessive daytime sleepiness.

Neuropathy: Risk factor for RLS involving affection of peripheral nerves.

Neurophysiological-neuroanatomical: One method of interpretation used by sleep scientists to explain the reasons why humans dream.

Neurotransmitter: Chemical responsible for transmitting nerve signals in the brain.

Night terror: Partial arousal disorder (like sleepwalking); also known as *pavor nocturnus.*

Nightmare: Vivid and frightening dreams, also known as dream anxiety attack.

Nocturnal eating/drinking syndrome: Condition characterized by awakening in the middle of the night, getting out of bed, and consuming large quantities of food quickly and uncontrollably, then returning to sleep.

Noradrenaline: One of the chemicals responsible for inactivation of REM sleep.

NREM: Non-rapid eye movement sleep. Multi-stage phase of the progression from wakefulness into deep sleep.

Obsessive-compulsive disorder: Condition characterized by repeated obsessions or intrusive thoughts and compulsions or repetitive compulsive behavior.

Owls: Group of people, called evening types, who go to sleep late and wake up late in the morning.

Pacemaker: Intrinsic biological clock located in the deeper part of the human brain which controls the rest-activity pattern.

Parkinson's disease (PD): A degenerative disorder of the central nervous system that often impairs the sufferer's motor skills and speech.

Partial arousal disorder: Condition in which the body is apparently active, but the brain is confused and only partially awakened.

Periodic limb movements in sleep (PLMS): Disorder characterized by periodic or semi-periodic movements of the limbs, mostly during NREM sleep.

Pillar procedure: Surgery on the palate in which polyester rods are implanted into the soft palate.

Pineal gland: Gland in the center of the brain which secretes melatonin.

Pituitary gland: The organ responsible for secretion of several important hormones.

Placebo: Inactive substance used in control experiment to reinforce a patient's expectation of obtaining result.

Platelets: Special types of blood cells involved in clot formation.

Poliomyelitis: Inflammation of the spinal cord, often called Infantile Paralysis.

Polyphasic sleep pattern: Alternating periods of 3 to 4 hours of sleep and waking observed in newborns.

Polysomnographic study: Overnight laboratory test used to diagnose primary sleep problems.

Postpolio syndrome: Weakness of arm or leg formerly affected by poliomyelitis, accompanied by paralysis of muscles including those of the previously unaffected extremities, and often breathing difficulties.

Postpolio syndrome: Weakness of arm or leg formerly affected by poliomyelitis, accompanied by paralysis of muscles and ofen breathing difficulties.

Predormitum: A state of diminished perception and control through which a person passes in progressing from wakefulness into the sleep state.

Premenstrual Syndrome: Condition, possibly caused by alterations in hormone levels, characterized by several negative symptoms including sleep difficulties similar to those of sleep deprivation.

Psychophysiologic insomnia: One type of insomnia for which a specific cause cannot be identified.

Rapid eye movement sleep behavior disorder (RBD): Dysfunction occurring in middle-aged to elderly people during REM sleep, characterized by dream enactment behavior.

REM: Rapid eye movement sleep. The stage of sleep during which dreaming occurs.

Restless Legs Syndrome (RLS): Common neurological and movement disorder characterized by intense disagreeable sensations and generally prevalent in the evening.

Retina: The layer of nerve cells at the back of the eye responsible for transmitting visual images to the back of the brain.

Rhythmic movement disorder: Benign condition, usually in infants younger than 18 months, and spontaneously outgrown. Sometimes confused with seizures occurring at night.

Serotonin: One of the chemicals responsible for inactivation of REM sleep.

Sleep apnea: Very serious sleep disturbing condition in which a sleeper stops breathing for at least 10 seconds several times during the night, resulting in interruptions of the sleep cycle.

Sleep deprivation: Condition of sleeplessness resulting in sleep debt and other adverse consequences.

Sleep latency: Is defined as the time elapsed between lights off and the first onset of any stage of sleep as determined by the changes in brain wave activity.

Sleep onset insomnia: Sleep disorder in which the patient is unable to fall asleep for long periods, resulting in insufficient rest and daytime tiredness.

Sleep paralysis: Feeling of paralysis of limbs and/or body at sleep onset or awakening from sleep.

Sleep related eating disorder (SRED): Type of sleep disorder in which people eat while in a state of partial arousal from sound sleep. They may eat in bed or roam through the house and prowl the kitchen.

Sleep spindles: Brain rhythms of 14 to 16 cycles per second that are seen in surface recordings taken from the front and center of the head during NREM sleep.

Snoring: Noisy sound generated by an obstruction to the free flow of air through the passages at the back of the mouth and nose caused by vibration of the uvula and soft palate during sleep, contributing to reduction of sleep quality.

Soft palate: Soft, muscular tissue in the back of the roof of the mouth.

Somnambulism: Sleepwalking. Very common in children, sometimes persisting into adulthood.

Spinal cord: Long tubular structure of the central nervous system that connects to the brain stem and runs through the vertebral column.

Sudden infant death syndrome (SIDS): Also known as crib death, the sudden death of an infant younger than one year of age, for which no cause is found.

Sundowning: Nocturnal confusion associated with partial or complete inversion of sleep rhythms.

Suprachiasmatic nuclei: Cluster of nerve cells within which the human internal clock is thought to reside.

Synapses: contact points between nerve cells in the brain.

Temporomandibular joint: The jaw joint.

Tolerance: Reduction in effect of a drug and need for higher doses to produce adequate effect.

Tonsils: Areas of lymphoid tissue on either side of the throat.

Transient insomnia: Also known as short-term or acute insomnia, resulting from an identifiable stressful situation.

Tricyclic antidepressants: Drugs having a 3-ring chemical structure.

Tryptophan: Serotonin precursor amino acid found in such foods as eggs, fish, bananas, peanuts and hard cheese, which modulates sleep.

Uvula: The small piece of soft pear-shaped structure that can be seen dan-gling down from the soft palate over the back of the tongue.

Video-polysomnographic study: Continuous video monitoring during a sleep study which measures physiological characteristics.

Zeitgebers: External time-givers removed during laboratory time-isolation experiments.

Index

Index